Springer-Verlag Wien GmbH

Acta Neurochirurgica
Supplements

Editor: H.-J. Steiger

Gamma Knife Radiosurgery

European Standards and Perspectives

Edited by
B. Wowra, J.-C. Tonn, and A. Muacevic

Acta Neurochirurgica
Supplement 91

Springer-Verlag Wien GmbH

PD. Dr. B. Wowra
Dr. A. Muacevic
German Gamma Knife Centre, Munich, Germany

Prof. Dr. J.-C. Tonn
Neurochirurgische Klinik und Poliklinik, Klinikum Großhadern, Munich, Germany

Originally published by Springer-Verlag / Wien in 2004
Softcover reprint of the hardcover 1st edition 2004

springeronline.com

Typesetting: Asco Typesetters, Hong Kong

Austria, www.theiss.at

Printed on acid-free and chlorine-free bleached paper

SPIN: 10998267

Library of Congress Control Number: 2004112956

With partly coloured Figures

ISSN 0065-1419
ISBN 978-3-7091-7200-1 ISBN 978-3-7091-0583-2 (eBook)
DOI 10.1007/978-3-7091-0583-2

Preface

The history of stereotactic radiosurgery dates back to more than 50 years. The concept was conceived by Lars Leksell already in 1951; in 1967 the first gamma knife was set up by Leksell. Since then Gamma Knife radiosurgery has grown continually in importance in recent years, both in terms of technological improvements and in terms of evaluation and broadening the treatment spectrum. Stereotactic radiosurgery of intracranial lesions is and will remain tightly interconnected with neurosurgery – not only in view of its history but also due to the fact that indication and risk assessment are always to be seen in the context of microneurosurgical alternative treatment. A crucial factor is that microneurosurgery and radiosurgery are not – as happened so often in the past – regarded as competing methods, even mutually excluding each other. This has led to fruitless controversies. Discussions of this method were directed by health care providers in this field towards an orientation disadvantageous for all concerned. Gamma Knife radiosurgery is a neurosurgical tool which may be used alone or in combination with microsurgery. Important is the neurosurgical know how to offer a safe and most effective treatment to the patient. For lesions treatable with just one technique at higher risk, therapy is often more effective and less invasive when the two treatment modalities are reasonably combined. Thus the medical and socioeconomic efficiency is equally increased.

In the present volume well-known European experts have defined their position on occasion of the 10-year anniversary of the German Gamma Knife Centre in Munich. This book gives an overview of the current status of European Gamma Knife radiosurgery. Leading European experts report on their specialities in Gamma Knife radiosurgery which is a state of the art summary of the possibilities and results of their current work. The book encompasses important as well as the more rare indications. All relevant technical and clinical quality standards are addressed. Only by continuously and prospectively evaluating the results of the radiosurgical and microneurosurgical therapy, in combination or alone, we will be in a position to offer to our patients the best individually adapted treatment strategy.

B. Wowra, J.-C. Tonn, and A. Muacevic

Acknowledgments

We gratefully acknowledge the professional help of Ilona Anders which made the timely publication of this book possible and the generous financial support of Electa company (Sweden) for the production of this volume.

Contents

Listed in Current Contents

Acta Neurochir (2004) [Suppl] 91: 1–7

Modern multimodal neuroimaging for radiosurgery: the example of PET scan integration

M. Levivier, N. Massager, D. Wikler, and **S. Goldman**

Neurosurgery & Gamma Knife Center, ULB Hôpital Erasme, Brussels, Belgium

Summary

Radiosurgery relies critically on medical imaging modalities. Leksell Gamma Knife® (LGK) radiosurgery presents the highest requirements in terms of imaging accuracy as the treatment is applied in a single high-dose session with no other spatial control than medical imaging. The advent of new imaging modalities opens challenges for LGK planning strategies. The integration of stereotactic PET in LGK represents an example of such application of modern multimodality imaging in radiosurgery. Our experience consists of 80 patients treated with the combination of MR/CT and PET guidance. In order to analyze the specific contribution of PET findings, we developed a classification reflecting the strategy used to define the target volume. When combining PET and MR information, 102 target volumes were defined, because some patients presented with multiple lesions or multifocal tumor areas. Abnormal PET uptake was found in 86% of the lesions, and this information altered significantly the MR-defined tumor in 73%. In conclusion, integration of PET in radiosurgery provides additional information opening new perspectives for the treatment of brain tumors. The use of a standardized classification allows to assess the relative role of PET. A similar approach could be useful and may serve as a template for the evaluation of the integration of other new imaging modalities in radiosurgery.

Keywords: Radiosurgery; gamma knife; functional imaging; PET.

Introduction

Radiosurgery treatment planning relies critically on medical imaging modalities. Medical images offer the ability to define a treatment target volume as well as a geometric transformation from the image space to the stereotactic frame space. Each modality likely to be used for image-guided therapy planning has to be validated for its clinical relevance and accuracy in order to be compatible with the application requirements. Leksell Gamma Knife® (LGK; Elekta Instruments A.B., Stockholm, Sweden) radiosurgery presents the highest requirements in terms of imaging and registration accuracy as the treatment is applied in a single high-dose session with no other spatial control than medical imaging. Until recently, the only proposed and validated imaging modalities for gamma knife radiosurgery treatment planning were 2D or 3D morphological representations of the brain such as x-ray ventriculography, computed tomography (CT), magnetic resonance (MR) imaging or digital subtraction angiography.

The advent of new functional imaging modalities such as positron emission tomography (PET), magnetic resonance spectroscopy, chemical shift imaging, diffusion and perfusion weighted magnetic resonance imaging, task-based activation, functional MRI maps, etc. along with the demonstration of their value either for highly specific and prognostic delineation of brain tumors or eloquent functional areas, opens new challenges for gamma knife radiosurgery planning strategies.

As a first step toward the integration of new imaging modalities in LGK radiosurgery, our personal experience is based on the validation and evaluation of the integration of stereotactic PET in the dosimetry planning [13]. The background of this approach is based on the previous experience with the use of PET in stereotactic conditions for brain biopsy [15]. Briefly, it shows that PET uptake is an accurate expression of the extent and of the degree of anaplasia in brain tumors. Moreover, for patients harboring tumors with similar histology, PET uptake is a significant indicator of the degree of aggressiveness and of the prognosis of survival. Thus, further integration of PET in neurosurgical procedures may contribute to a better management of brain tumors, either in optimizing the delineation of their extension, or in defining the aggressive areas of heterogeneous large tumors. This strategy has been initiated with the integration of PET metabolic information in the neurosurgical planning of brain tumor resection using neuronavigation [14]. Accordingly, when we started with LGK radiosurgery, it was a logical step to also integrate PET in this therapeutic approach. In the following, our clinical experience with patients that have undergone LGK radiosurgery guided by the combination of MR/CT and PET stereotactic images is summarized.

Materials and methods

Between December 1999 and January 2004, 80 patients had stereotactic PET as part of their image acquisition for the planning of LGK radiosurgery. Standard preparation was similar for all our patients undergoing LGK radiosurgery. Briefly, the Leksell G frame (Elekta Instruments A.B., Stockholm, Sweden) was attached to the patient's head under local anesthesia with mild sedation (except in the pediatric population, where the entire radiosurgical procedure is performed under general anesthesia). Stereotactic CT was always acquired as a standard quality control for MR distortion and PET threshold. Stereotactic MR was obtained using different images acquisition parameters, depending on the nature and the location of the lesion. T1-weighted images before and after intravenous injection of gadolinium-diethylenetriaminepentaacetic acid (Gd-DTPA) was, however, obtained in all patients in this series with stereotactic PET, and was used as the primary reference for target definition on MR. In this particular group, the patients were then transferred to the PET/Biomedical Cyclotron Unit, which is directly connected to the main hospital building and to the gamma knife Center.

Stereotactic PET images were acquired with the Siemens/CTI ECAT 962 (HR+) 2D and 3D tomograph (Knoxville, Tennessee), allowing simultaneous acquisition of 63 planes with a slice thickness of 2.4 mm. This high precision PET imager is now used for all our stereotactic procedures. PET image acquisition with the Leksell G frame has been validated using a 3D Lucite phantom containing spherical simulated targets that can be imaged both in PET and CT and provides sub-millimetric spatial accuracy [13]. The PET image files in the CTI ECAT 7 proprietary format are transferred to the Hewlett-Packard workstation used for treatment planning with Leksell GammaPlan® (LGP; Elekta Instruments A.B., Stockholm, Sweden). A custom software converting the PET data file format to the LGP file format is used to import PET images. The PET volume is then handled as a CT or MR volume in LGP, and therefore accessible only for visualization in a linear gray scale. To allow the analysis of PET images with a high contrast pseudo colour lookup table (LUT), we replace the gray scale LUT file with our own PET colour LUT file. The integration of PET image modality in LGP is an ongoing project in collaboration with Elekta R&D department. The current PET software module is not a commercially available version, and its clinical evaluation is performed in the framework of a protocol approved by the Ethics Committee of our institution.

Once defined in LGP, the stereotactic PET images are correlated with the other stereotactic image modalities of the same patient and can be used for determination of the target volume. The planning always begins with a separate analysis of each *stereotactic image modality*. A 3-D volumetric contour is drawn on the stereotactic MR, on the basis of the neuroradiologic definition of the tumor, on the diagnostic images; for radiosurgery, this mostly corresponds to the delineation of the area of Gd-DTPA enhancement. Then, the stereotactic PET images are analyzed independently of the MR images, jointly by the nuclear medicine physician, the neurosurgeon, and the radiation therapist. Both gray scale as well as pseudo-colour LUT images are used. Abnormal metabolism suitable for target definition corresponds either to areas of increased tracer uptake as compared to the surrounding normal appearing brain or to foci of relative increase of the tracer in a hypometabolic lesion. A 3-D volumetric PET contour delineating these areas is drawn on a visual basis or using the software-based segmentation algorithm, and is projected onto the corresponding MR images. The final target volume is defined and drawn on the stereotactic MR taking into account the respective contributions of PET and MR as well as the anatomical location of the tumor and the functional areas at risk.

In order to analyze the specific contribution of PET as compared to MR in the definition of the target volume, we have developed classification that reflects the strategy used to define the target volume [11]. Briefly, the description of the relative location of the projection of PET and MR volumes is considered first, yielding 6 classes (*class I*: PET-defined volume projects within the MR-defined volume; *class II*: PET- and MR-defined volumes do not fully project in the same areas; *class III*: MR-defined volume projects within PET-defined volume; *class IV*: PET- and MR-defined volumes are similar; *class V*: a PET volume can be defined but MR is not contributive (no contrast enhancement or non-specific signal changes); *class VI*: an MR volume can be defined, but PET is not contributive because there is no specific uptake area that can be contoured). Based on these categories, a choice is made secondarily to define the target volume when PET and MR volumes are different. Thus, in classes I, II and III, different sub-groups (noted A, B, and C, respectively) can be defined if only PET-, only MR-, or a combination of the PET- and MR-defined volumes are used to define the target volume. For classes IV to VI, however, there is only one definition of target volume and no sub-groups are used. Based on this classification, usefulness of the PET findings may be evaluated [11]. The contribution of PET is considered valuable (i.e. the target volume is significantly altered, based on PET information) in classes I.A. and I.B., II.A. and II.B., III.A. and III.B., and V.

Results

Stereotactic PET images were successfully acquired, transferred to LGP and integrated in the dosimetry planning of all patients. PET in stereotactic conditions was easily performed, within a 90-minute period, and did not cause any major additional discomfort to the patient.

For these 80 treatment sessions, the patients were offered LGK radiosurgery with PET guidance (LGK-PET) because their tumor was ill-defined on MR and we anticipated some limitation of target definition on MR alone. This represents more or less 10% of the total number of LGK radiosurgery procedures performed in our center during the same period of time. LGK-PET was used in the following indications: 48 primary CNS lesions (60%), 16 recurrent metastases (20%), and 16 pituitary adenomas (20%). We used 2 different radiotracers: ^{18}F-FDG was chosen in 33 patients (41%), and ^{11}C-methionine in 47 patients (59%). When combining stereotactic PET and MR information in LGP, 102 target volumes were defined for the 80 LGK-PET treatment sessions because patients presented with multiple lesions or multifocal tumor areas. The analysis is based on the 102 target volumes (and not the 80 patients) because some targets in the same patient have different PET and MR characteristics, *yielding to* different strategies in defining the target volumes.

Altogether, for the 102 targets, there were 62 target volumes in the primary CNS tumors, 24 in the metastases, and 16 in the pituitary adenomas. The volume of PET uptake projected within the MR-defined tumor (class I) in 37 targets (36% of all LGK-PET). In more than half of these cases, the target volume was based primarily on the PET information. Abnormal PET and MR areas *projected*, at least partially, in different regions (class II) for 26 targets (25% of all LGK-PET). The target volume was based primarily on PET information (useful PET) in 23 cases, either because the target volume was restricted to the area of PET uptake, or because the target volume combined and included the entire PET and MR abnormal areas. The MR-defined volume was smaller and projected into a larger PET-defined volume (class III) in 7 targets (7% of all LGK-PET). The target volume was based on PET and included the entire PET volume in 6 of them. PET was not specifically used for target definition when PET- and MR-defined volumes were similar (class IV) in 5 targets (5% of all LGK-PET). Finally, the area of increased PET uptake was used as the sole information to define the target volume because MR was considered not contributive (class V) in 14 targets (14% of all LGK-PET) and there was no specific PET uptake and the target volume had to be defined on MR only (class VI) in 14 targets (14%).

Altogether (Fig. 1), abnormal PET uptake (all classes, except class VI) was found in 88 of the 102 lesions (86%). In these 88 lesions, the information obtained from stereotactic PET contributed to the definition of the target volume in altering significantly the MR-defined volume in 64 targets (73% of all positive PET). Two representative examples are shown in Fig. 2. We have noticed differences in the contribution of PET among the clinical indications. PET was considered useful in 76% of the primary CNS tumors, in 68% of the metastases, and in 60% of the pituitary adenomas.

Discussion

Both technically and clinically, the use of PET for radiosurgery is a continuation of our previous work on the integration of metabolic information in image-guided neurosurgery [14]. Here, the results also confirm that PET contains metabolic information that are independent of the morphological information provided by CT or MR and that the integration of PET images in neurosurgical approaches, including radiosurgery, is useful for the management of brain tumors. Interestingly, similar approaches have recently been reported for the radiotherapy planning of gliomas with ^{123}I-α-methyl-tyrosine-SPECT [7] and with PET with ^{18}F-FDG [19].

From a technical point of view, registration of PET images to other modalities for the treatment of patients may be considered in the context of frame-based high precision procedures, such as stereotactic biopsy, frame-based open surgery or radiosurgery as well as in the context of frameless procedures such as neuronavigation or radiotherapy. The choice of one or the other approach relies on a trade-off between accuracy and reliability against minimal invasiveness and clinical routine feasibility. For stereotactic PET, as it was used here for LGK radiosurgery, an imaging fiducials system defining the stereotactic coordinate space of the frame attached to the patient is no doubt the most accurate and reliable way of registering PET images with patient treatment space. Nevertheless, this requires careful solutions in addressing the various technical challenges associated with PET acquisition, as discussed in detail elsewhere [12]. Phantom based validation has been conducted to verify the application accuracy of the procedure [9], and the figures for mean and maximum fiducial registration error provide a valid indicator for stereotactic PET accuracy. In our experience, fiducial registration mean error is around 0.2 mm of mean for the volume, with a maximum value around 0.6 mm for higher error slice. Frameless PET should also be considered for the management of these patients, either in the context of a better evaluation of the follow-up PET examinations or as a tentative alternative to stereotactic PET for radiosurgery planning. The frameless approach may have the advantage to extend accessibility to PET in radiosurgery to a larger number of centers. Comfort and planning flexibility would also benefit from the non-invasiveness of the procedure. This requires solutions to register PET without frame fiducials yet with high accuracy

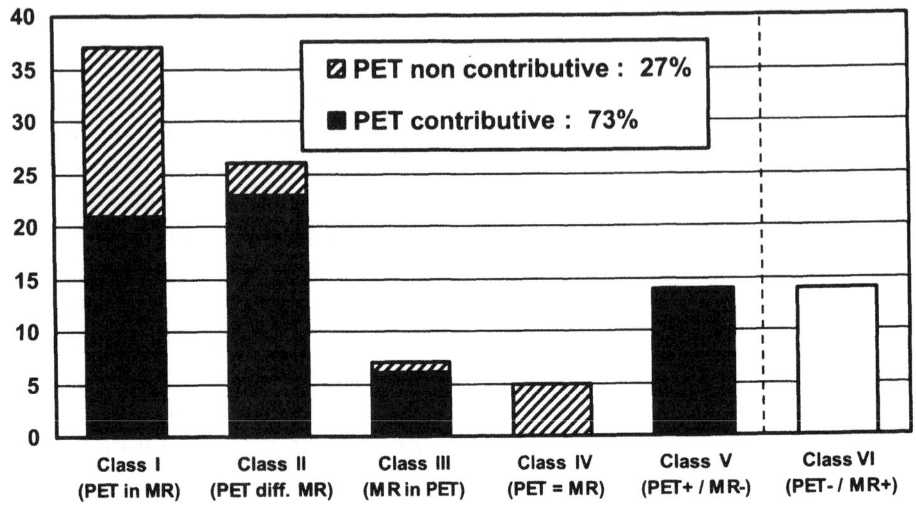

Fig. 1. Distribution of 102 lesions according to the proposed classification of the relative PET and MR contribution to the definition of the target volume in each of the 6 classes

and reliability and we currently perform studies to evaluate the feasibility and reliability of integrating frameless PET in LGK radiosurgery [21].

Compared to our experience with PET-guided stereotactic biopsy or neuronavigation, the use of LGK-PET has generated its own therapeutic challenges in relation with the specific planning requirements of this approach. Stereotactic biopsy is a limited neurosurgical procedure for which stereotactic PET may play a role for the selection of a discrete target [10]. Therefore, target selection will not be hindered by extensive PET abnormalities. On the contrary, stereotactic PET will help to optimize it, aiming at sampling the most representative area of the tumor [10, 16, 17]. Also with neuronavigation, even when stereotactic PET anomalies cannot be fully incorporated into the final target volume, standard cytoreductive surgery based on anatomical landmarks is the alternative, and the comparison between pre-operative and post-operative PET will help to objectively evaluate the extent of tumor resection [3]. Even in those cases information provided by PET are used to further evaluate the prognosis and the need for adjuvant therapies [2, 4]. In radiosurgery, however, the limitation in the treatable target volume requires a strict strategy for the selection of the patients that may benefit from LGK-PET, as well as for the *a priori* choice of radiotracer and target definition. This is especially important when using LGK-PET in infiltrating brain tumors or for lesions that are not well defined on MR, in order to avoid circumstances where stereotactic PET images show an extended uptake of the radiotracer that is incompatible with radiosurgery, requiring to abort the procedure. Also, at the time of planning, an assumption has to be made about the relevance of the presence of tumor tissue in the entire area of increased PET tracer uptake. Indeed, image-based radiosurgical plannings do not allow documentation of histology to confirm that either PET- or MR-defined tumor volumes are correct. Such data, correlating MR findings with histology, have been obtained with stereotactic biopsies of brain tumors [8]. Along the same line, our long-term experience of the correlation of the pathology of stereotactic biopsy with their metabolic characteristics [5, 6], as well as the increased knowledge about PET in brain tumor in the literature [22] strengthen the valuable link between PET uptake and histology in brain tumors. Moreover, the clinical context, with most patients in our series harboring recurrent tumors (with known histology from previous surgery) or inoperable tumors (with known histology from stereotactic biopsy or from a primary tumor), also limits the risk of erroneous target selection using combined PET and MR data. Of course, one cannot rule out that some PET areas that have been included in target volumes could have contained necrotic non tumorous tissue, especially when treating recurrent malignant gliomas after radiation therapy or recurrent metastases after previous radiosurgery. Recent papers addressing this issue also support the use of PET in

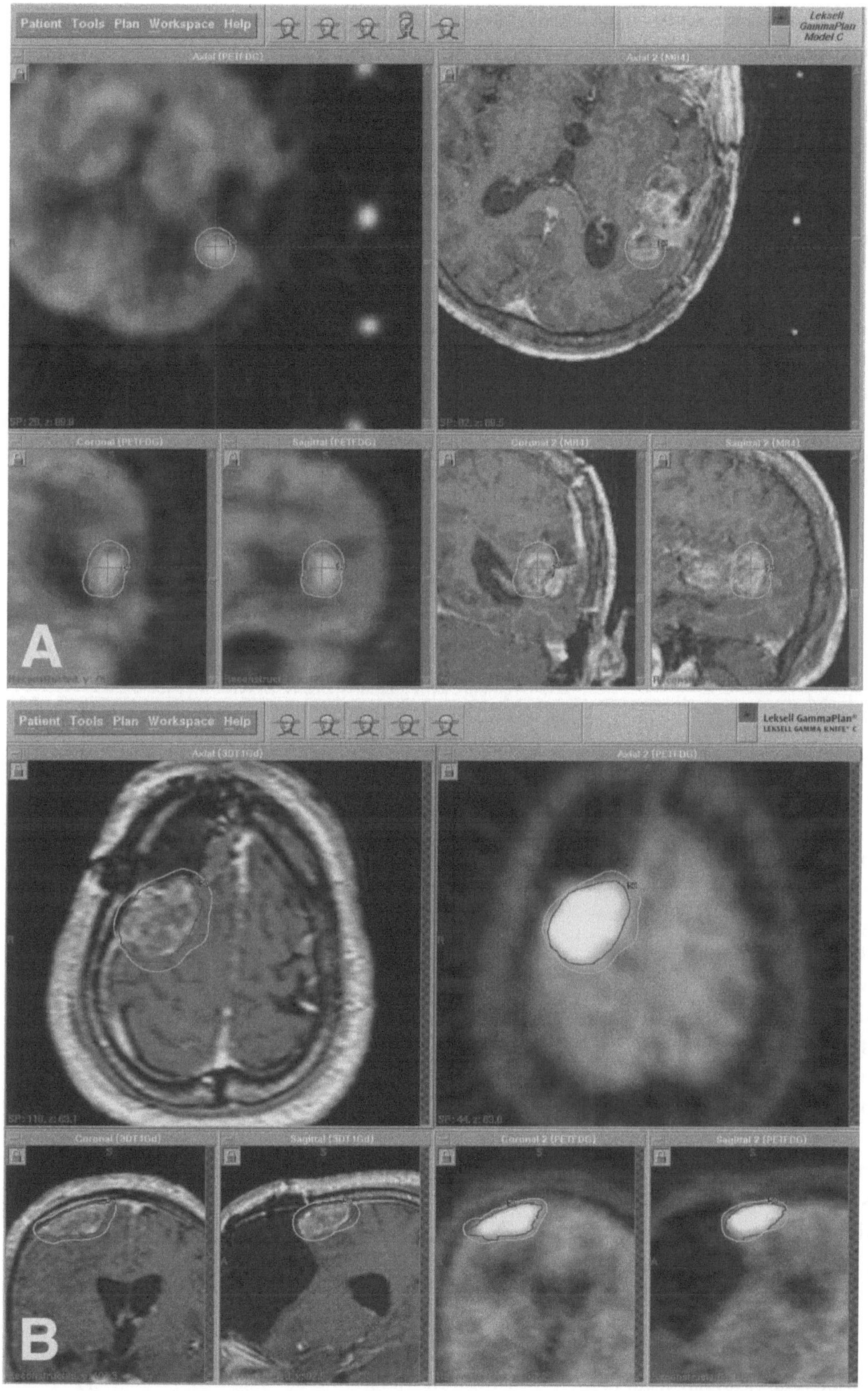

Fig. 2. Example of combined MR and PET guidance with ^{18}F-FDG in 2 patients with recurrent glioblastoma. (A) PET images (left side) allowed to define an area of hypermetabolism, which corresponded only to the posterior part of the gadolinium enhancement when projected on MR (right side). Only this area was used as the target volume and encompassed in the prescription isodose volume. (B) PET images (right side) showed a large area of increased tracer uptake; when projected on the corresponding MR (right side), this volume corresponded to the entire area of gadolinium enhancement and was used as the target volume to define the prescription isodose volume

those conditions [1, 19, 20]. Also, we believe that complementary investigations, such as with MR spectroscopy, may be of important help in that respect [18].

The possibility to use and to integrate stereotactic PET in the dosimetry planning for LGK radiosurgery provides a unique opportunity to evaluate the benefit of this procedure and its scope of application in radiosurgery. However, its real clinical advantage needs a comparative evaluation of local tumor control, functional results, and survival for the different clinical indications. For better objective evaluation of the benefits of the procedure we developed a descriptive classification illustrating the relative information provided by PET and MR [11]. Two steps are used. Firstly, the description of the relative location of the projection of the PET and MR volumes is considered, *yielding* 6 classes. Secondly, the choice in defining the final target volume may *yield to* 3 sub-groups, depending on the amount of PET and MR volumes that are included. As this classification has been used to record and categorize the strategy of each treatment planning, it has proven to be useful for the assessment of the role of stereotactic PET. Moreover, it allowed to group and identify classes corresponding to different planning strategies with PET. Indeed, in some instances, MR disclosed a large abnormal volume that was not compatible with LGK radiosurgery, and PET was used to focus the treatment on the metabolic active part of the tumor. Conversely, in some cases, the target volume was maximized thanks to the use of PET, and the delineation of the treated tumor would have been underestimated if MR only was used. Again, the real benefit for the patients will need further long-term analysis of the clinical results. We also believe that further accumulation of prospective data using this classification will allow to better distinguish the type of contribution PET provides in relation with the different clinical indications. Similarly, this approach could be useful and may serve as a template for the evaluation of the integration of other new functional imaging modalities in radiosurgery.

References

1. Belohlávek O, Simonova G, Kantorova I, Novotny J, Jr., Liscák R (2003) Brain metastases after stereotactic radiosurgery using the Leksell gamma knife: can FDG PET help to differentiate radionecrosis from tumour progression? Eur J Nucl Med 30: 96–100
2. De Witte O, Goldberg I, Wikler D, Rorive S, Damhaut P, Monclus M, Salmon I, Brotchi J, Goldman S (2001) Positron emission tomography with injection of methionine as a prognostic factor in glioma. J Neurosurg 95: 746–750
3. De Witte O, Levivier M, Violon P, Brotchi J, Goldman S (1998) Quantitative imaging study of extent of surgical resection and prognosis of malignant astrocytomas. Neurosurgery 43: 398–399
4. De Witte O, Levivier M, Violon P, Salmon I, Damhaut P, Wikler D, Jr., Hildebrand J, Brotchi J, Goldman S (1996) Prognostic value of positron emission tomography with [18F]fluoro-2-deoxy-D-glucose in the low-grade glioma. Neurosurgery 39: 470–476
5. Goldman S, Levivier M, Pirotte B, Brucher JM, Wikler D, Damhaut P, Stanus E, Brotchi J, Hildebrand J (1996) Regional glucose metabolism and histopathology of gliomas – A study based on positron emission tomography-guided stereotactic biopsy. Cancer 78: 1098–1106
6. Goldman S, Levivier M, Pirotte B, Brucher J-M, Wikler D, Damhaut P, Dethy S, Brotchi J, Hildebrand J (1997) Regional methionine and glucose metabolism in gliomas: a comparative study on PET-guided stereotactic biopsy. J Nucl Med 38: 1–4
7. Grosu AL, Feldmann H, Dick S, Dzewas B, Nieder C, Gumprecht H, Frank A, Schwaiger M, Molls M, Weber WA (2002) Implications of IMT-SPECT for postoperative radiotherapy planning in patients with gliomas. Int J Radiat Oncol Biol Phys 54: 842–854
8. Kelly PJ, Daumas-Duport C, Scheithauer BW, Kall BA, Kispert DB (1987) Stereotactic histologic correlations of computed tomography- and resonance imaging-defined abnormalities in patients with glial neoplasms. Mayo Clin Proc 62: 450–459
9. Levivier M, Goldman S, Bidaut LM, Luxen A, Stanus E, Przedborski S, Balériaux D, Hildebrand J, Brotchi J (1992) Positron emission tomography-guided stereotactic brain biopsy. Neurosurgery 31: 792–797
10. Levivier M, Goldman S, Pirotte B, Brucher J-M, Balériaux D, Luxen A, Hildebrand J, Brotchi J (1995) Diagnostic yield of stereotactic brain biopsy guided by positron emission tomography with [18F]fluorodeoxyglucose. J Neurosurg 82: 445–452
11. Levivier M, Massager N, Wikler D, Lorenzoni J, Ruiz S, Devriendt D, David P, Desmedt F, Simon S, Van Houtte P, Brotchi J, Goldman S (2004) The use of stereotactic PET images in the dosimetry planning of radiosurgery for brain tumors: Clinical experience and proposed classification. J Nucl Med 45: 1146–1154
12. Levivier M, Wikler D, De Witte O, Massager N, Goldman S, Brotchi J (2003) Positron Emission Tomography (PET) for the Management of Brain Tumors. In: Black PM, Loeffler J (eds) Cancer of the Nervous System, 2nd edn (in press)
13. Levivier M, Wikler D, Goldman S, David P, Metens T, Massager N, Gerosa M, Devriendt D, Desmedt F, Simon S, Van Houtte P, Brotchi J (2000) Integration of the metabolic data of positron emission tomography in the dosimetry planning of radiosurgery with the gamma knife: early experience with brain tumors. J Neurosurg 93 [Suppl] 3: 233–238
14. Levivier M, Wikler D, Goldman S, Pirotte B, Brotchi J (1999) Positron emission tomography in stereotactic conditions as a functional imaging technique for neurosurgical guidance. In: Alexander III EB, Maciunas RM (eds) Advanced neurosurgical navigation. Thieme Medical Publishers, New York, pp 85–99
15. Levivier M, Wikler D, Jr., Massager N, David P, Devriendt D, Lorenzoni J, Pirotte B, Desmedt F, Simon S, Jr, Goldman S, Van Houtte P, Brotchi J (2002) The integration of metabolic imaging in stereotactic procedures including radiosurgery: a review. J Neurosurg 97: 542–550
16. Massager N, David P, Goldman S, Pirotte B, Wikler D, Salmon

I, Nagy N, Brotchi J, Levivier M (2000) Combined magnetic resonance imaging- and positron emission tomography-guided stereotactic biopsy in brainstem mass lesions: diagnostic yield in a series of 30 patients. J Neurosurg 93: 951–957
17. Pirotte B, Goldman S, Salzberg S, Wikler D, David P, Vandesteene A, Van Bogaert P, Salmon I, Brotchi J, Levivier M (2003) Combined positron emission tomography and magnetic resonance imaging for the planning of stereotactic brain biopsies in children: experience in 9 cases. Pediatr Neurosurg 38: 146–155
18. Rock JP, Hearshen D, Scarpace L, Croteau D, Gutierrez J, Fisher JL, Rosenblum ML, Mikkelsen T (2002) Correlations between magnetic resonance spectroscopy and image-guided histopathology, with special attention to radiation necrosis. Neurosurgery 51: 912–919
19. Tralins KS, Douglas JG, Stelzer KJ, Mankoff DA, Silbergeld DL, Rostomilly R, Hummel S, Scharnhorst J, Krohn KA, Spence AM (2002) Volumetric analysis of 18F-FDG PET in glioblastoma multiforme: prognostic information and possible role in definition of target volumes in radiation dose escalation. J Nucl Med 43: 1667–1673
20. Tsuyuguchi N, Sunada I, Iwai Y, Yamanaka K, Tanaka K, Takami T, Otsuka Y, Sakamoto S, Ohata K, Goto T, Hara M (2003) Methionine positron emission tomography of recurrent metastatic brain tumor and radiation necrosis after stereotactic radiosurgery: is a differential diagnosis possible? J Neurosurg 98: 1056–1064
21. Wikler D, Sadeghi N, Goldman S, Massager N, Levivier M (2004) Clinical validation methodology for the use of frameless PET in Leksell gamma knife® radiosurgery. Radiosurgery 5: 247–254
22. Wong TZ, van der Westhuizen GJ, and Coleman RE (2002) Positron emission tomography imaging of brain tumors. Neuroimag Clin N Am 12: 615–626

Correspondence: Marc Levivier, M.D., Ph.D., Neurosurgery & Gamma Knife Center, U.L.B. – Hôpital Erasme, 808, route de Lennik, 1070 Brussels, Belgium. e-mail: Marc.Levivier@ulb.ac.be

Acta Neurochir (2004) [Suppl] 91: 9–23

High precision radiosurgery and technical standards

S. G. Scheib[1], **S. Gianolini**[1], **N. J. Lomax**[1], and **A. Mack**[2]

[1] Department of Medical Radiation Physics, Klinik Im Park, Zurich, Switzerland
[2] Gamma Knife Centre Frankfurt, Frankfurt, Germany

Summary

Background. A high degree of precision and accuracy in radiosurgery is a fundamental requirement for therapeutic success. Small radiation fields and steep dose gradients are clinically applied thus necessitating a dedicated quality assurance program in order to guarantee dosimetric and geometric accuracy.

Material and methods. A detailed analysis of the course of treatment independent of the irradiation technique used results in the so-called chain of uncertainties in radiosurgery (immobilisation, imaging, treatment planning system, definition of regions of interest, mechanical accuracy, dose planning, dose verification). Each link in this chain is analysed for accuracy and the established quality assurance procedures are discussed. A "System Test" was used to check the whole chain of uncertainties simultaneously.

Results. The tests described are compatible with published reports on quality assurance in radiosurgery. In terms of accuracy the weakest link in the chain of uncertainties is stereotactic MR imaging. Geometric overall accuracy measured in the "System Test" is less than 0.7 mm.

Conclusion. The established quality assurance routines have clinically been validated. MR imaging dominates geometric overall accuracy in radiosurgery, which can be limited to less than 1 mm by an adequate quality assurance protocol.

Keywords: Radiosurgery; gamma knife; quality assurance; System Test.

Introduction

Stereotactic radiosurgery (SRS) refers to non-invasive precise irradiation of small (volume typically less than 25 cm^3), clearly circumscribed, stereotactically defined lesions. Stereotactic means precise, three-dimensional localisation of anatomical structures (within the brain) using diagnostic imaging modalities. SRS is performed by cross-firing collimated narrow beams of ionizing radiation such as heavy charged particles (protons, alpha-particles, heavier ions), x-rays or gamma radiation. In contrast to conventional radiation therapy or fractionated stereotactically guided radiation therapy (SRT), a high radiation dose is given in a single session in SRS. To avoid side effects in radiosurgery, normal tissue sparing which is usually achieved by low dose fractionation must be compensated for by a corresponding lower dose to normal tissue. This prerequisite for a complication free lesion control must be achieved in SRS by a high degree of geometric dose application accuracy combined with highly conformal dose distributions.

Today SRS is performed using either protons available in dedicated facilities only, x-rays produced by adapted linear accelerators (linac), or gamma rays in the case of gamma knife® [1, 7, 19]. Common to all these techniques is the use of narrow collimated beams directed towards the target from several directions in order to concentrate the dose within the target and to blur the dose in the surrounding normal tissue. These irradiation techniques usually produce small fields (full width at half maximum – FWHM – down to 4 mm) and steep dose gradients (up to 40% per mm). Thus dedicated quality assurance protocols must be applied in order to guarantee an accurate treatment. Today, in the case of adapted linacs, not only circular shaped x-ray beams are used but also small irregular fields shaped by a micromultileaf collimator mounted to or integrated in the linac in order to fit the irregular target outline seen in the beams' eye view [2, 3].

Quality assurance in SRS (and SRT) is of utmost importance and is one of the tasks of medical physicists in charge of a clinical SRS/SRT program. In the literature several contributions can be found addressing this issue [6, 13, 15–18, 20, 23, 26]. Since the course of radiosurgical treatment is rather independent of the treatment unit itself, the quality assurance components addressed here are applicable to different irradiation techniques. Considering that the authors' experience in radiosurgery to a high degree is based on the gamma knife®, this treatment unit is described in more detail. Also, the majority of patients to date (more than 260'000), suffering from meningiomas, CPA schwannomas, arterio-venous malformations (AVMs), pituitary adenomas, brain metastases, glial tumours, trigeminal neuralgia, etc., have been treated by approximately 200 gamma knife® centres world wide.

Materials and methods

The gamma knife®

The gamma knife® unit (Fig. 1a) consists of a cast iron housing containing 201 cobalt 60 sources in a semi-hemispherical arrangement delivering their gamma radiation to the corresponding 201 fixed primary beam channels. The patient couch (sliding cradle) supports the exchangeable final collimator system (collimator helmet). A cross sectional view of the gamma knife® with the patient couch in treatment position is shown in Fig. 1b, and a single beam channel is shown in Fig. 1c. The 201 beams are arranged in 5 rings on a semi-hemispherical surface which leads to rotationally symmetrical dose distributions in the patients' long axis.

The collimator system is designed as to produce a precise overlap of the 201 individual beam axes at the mechanical isocentre, the unit centre point (UCP) of the gamma knife®. There are four designated collimator helmets 4, 8, 14 and 18 mm, (Fig. 2a), these being the FWHM of the dose profile for a single beam at the UCP. The superposition of all 201 beams, schematically shown in figure 2b, then produces almost spherically shaped dose distributions with slightly increased FWHM dimensions of 6, 11, 19 and 24 mm (in x- and y-directions) respectively at the isocentre (Fig. 2c). In Fig. 3 relative dose profiles along the y-axis are shown for the four collimator helmets, measured with dosimeters appropriate for small field photon dosimetry [17], which where shifted within a 16 cm diameter spherical polystyrene phantom placed at the isocentre of the unit ($x = y = z = 100.0$ mm).

Each dose application resulting in a near spherical dose distribution is usually called a shot or an isocentre. Several such shots, typically using different collimator helmets, need to be distributed throughout the lesion volume in order to cover three dimensional irregular shaped lesions with a given prescription isodose [28]. This multi-isocentric dose planning procedure is able to cover the whole lesion with the prescription isodose, including regions of increased dose within the target due to the effect of overlapping shots causing nonhomogeneous dose distributions within the target. In Fig. 4 an example of an outlined target volume for a pituitary adenoma (prolactinoma) is shown in axial, coronal and sagittal views (top row from left to right) together with the optic tract outlined as a region of interest (ROI). The overlapping shots for this multi-isocentric dose planning using five 8 mm and eight 4 mm collimator helmets are shown in the middle row of Fig. 4. The bottom row of Fig. 4 shows the resultant dose distribution which is optimised in such a way as to cover the lesion with at least the 50% isodose line, which in this case was 25 Gy. The dose distribution is normalised to the dose maximum (100%) lying within the target. The lower isodose line (16%) in Fig. 4 indicates the 8 Gy isodose line, which is recognised as the tolerance dose for the optic tract. Note the rapid dose fall-off toward the optic tract which enables treatment of lesions located close to critical structures.

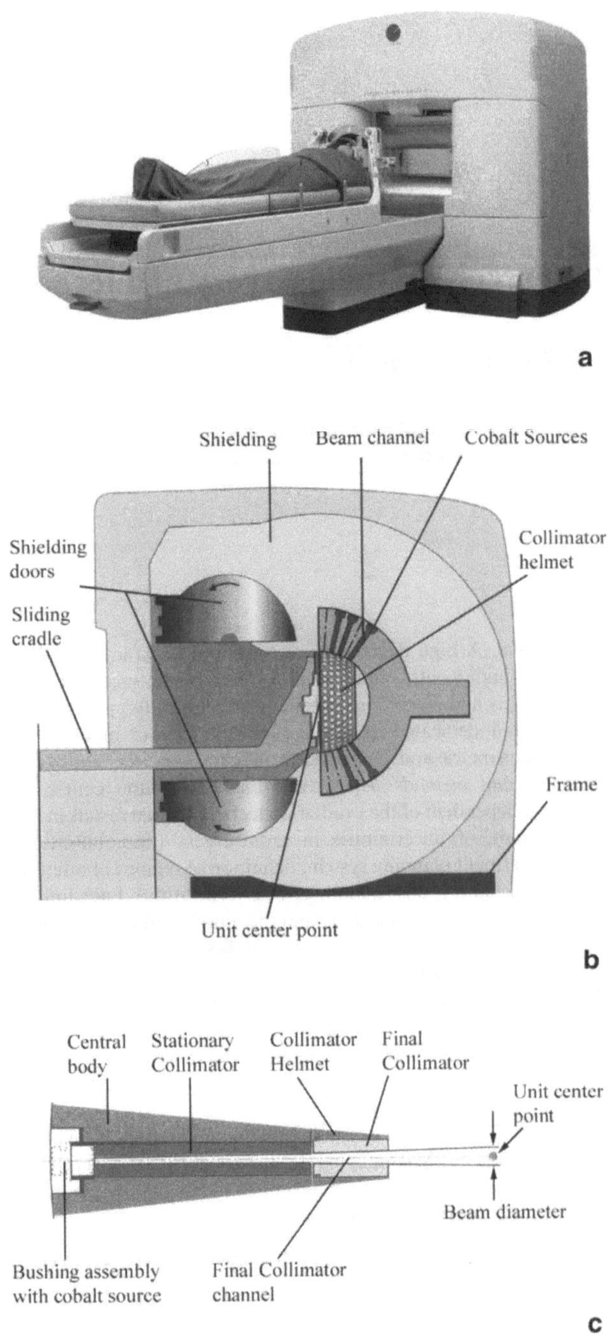

Fig. 1. (a) Photograph of the gamma knife® C consisting of the radiation shielding in the back and the patient couch in the front (Courtesy of Elekta Instrument AB). (b) Cross sectional view of the gamma knife® with the patient couch in treatment position (Courtesy of Elekta Instrument AB). (c) One of the 201 single beam channels of the gamma knife® (Courtesy of Elekta Instrument AB)

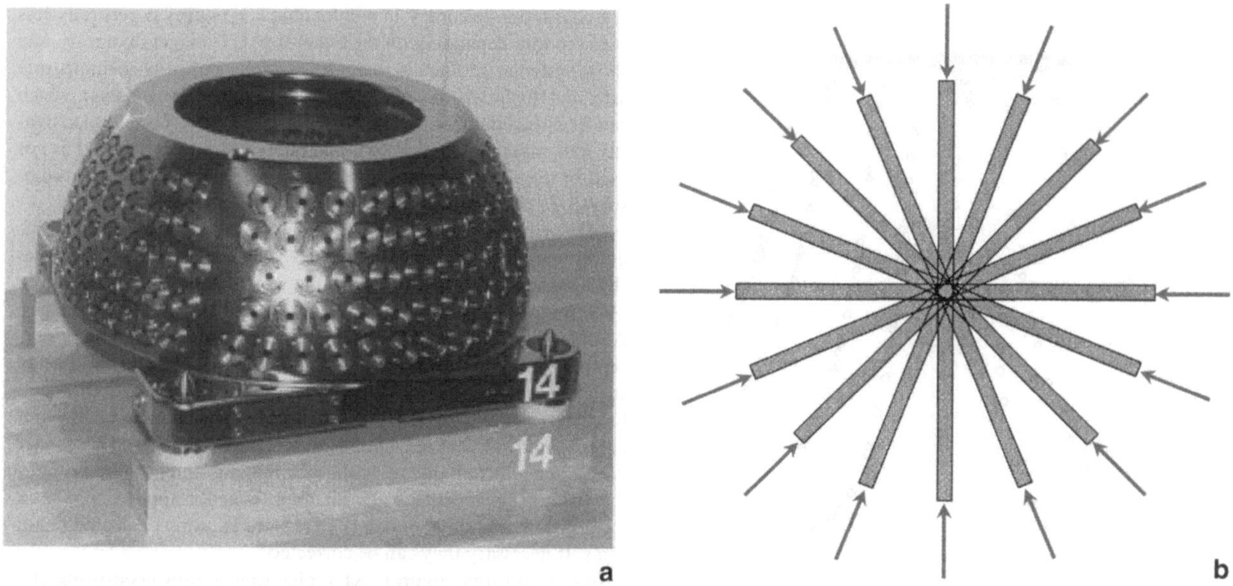

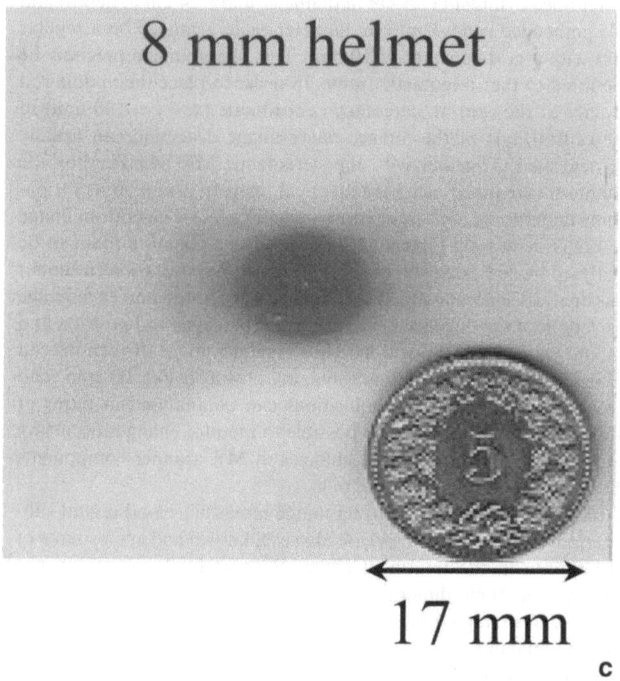

Fig. 2. (a) Photograph of one of the four collimator helmets (14 mm beam diameter at isocentre) for the gamma knife®, fitted with 201 final collimators defining the beam diameter. (b) Schematic drawing representing the superposition of the simultaneous incident beams (cross firing) which intersect at the unit centre point (UCP) of the gamma knife®. (c) Radiochromic film measurement of the resultant two dimensional dose distribution for the 8 mm collimator helmet in the x-y-plane of the stereotactic coordinate system

The chain of uncertainties

One reason for a successful radiosurgical treatment is the geometrically accurate placement of a defined dose including the steep dose gradient in the patient by applying precisely defined procedures starting from placement of the stereotactic frame through to dose verification. Owing to the small field sizes, the high dose, the high degree of conformity, and the small safety margins applied, leading to an increased risk of target underdosage and/or normal tissue overdosage in SRS, accuracy and precision, monitored by a quality assurance and control protocol, is of utmost importance. Precision refers to the reproducibility of a measurement based on the results of repeated measurements without changing procedure and instrumentation. Standard deviation of the measured values provide a measure of consistency of the procedure applied, but when discussing precision no information on the agreement with the "true" value is given. In contrast, accuracy denotes the closeness of agreement between the "true" and the measured value and includes systemic errors. A possible inaccuracy refers directly to systemic errors in the measured procedure and requires special attention.

For quality assurance procedures the treatment is separated into its different components, visualised by a so-called chain of uncertainties as shown in Fig. 5. After the stereotactic immobilisation (a) of the patient's head, stereotactic imaging (b) is then necessary to

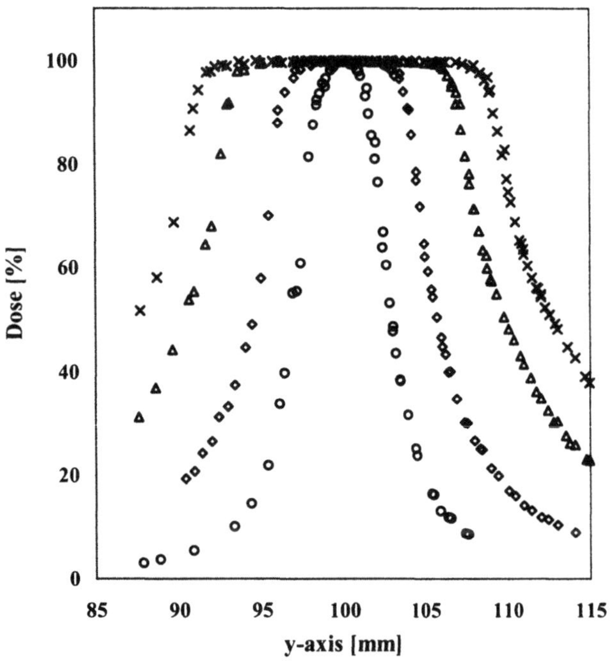

Fig. 3. Measured relative dose profiles along the y-axis for the 4 mm (circles), 8 mm (diamonds), 14 mm (triangles) and 18 mm (crosses) collimator helmet using all 201 beams

define the stereotactic space and to delineate the target and relevant ROIs (d) using the treatment planning system (c). Furthermore the mechanical accuracy (e) of the treatment unit has to be checked and the accuracy limits of the dose calculation (f) as implemented in the treatment planning system have to be known. Finally dose verifications (g) are performed in order to compare calculated and measured dose distributions. In addition to checking each link in this chain, a so-called "System Test" is also of help to manage the whole chain of uncertainties in a single experiment. A quality assurance tool of more clinical relevance is the volumetric follow up (h) of the lesions treated.

Stereotactic immobilisation

The stereotactic Leksell frame shown in Fig. 6 defines the stereotactic coordinate system. This Cartesian coordinate system has its origin at the right posterior top position indicated. The frame is fixed under local anaesthesia with the help of skull fixation pins and guarantees sub-millimetre positioning accuracy during imaging and treatment. Relocatable fixation systems, usually masks, are less accurate.

Stereotactic imaging

It is well known that stereotactic imaging modalities show systematic inaccuracies in target point localisation which require special attention. Conventional x-ray imaging does not demonstrate systemic image distortions, therefore, when using this imaging modality, localisation accuracy of known target points is dominated by the precision of the method and typically lies in the range of about 0.2 mm.

Localisation accuracy in stereotactic CT images is generally less than 0.6 mm depending on the voxel size. CT images do not usually show systemic geometric image distortions but often demonstrate artefacts (high density streak and beam hardening artefacts), which can be disturbing from a diagnostic point of view. The electron density information (Hounsfield units) offered by a calibrated CT is not used in the dose calculation for arc based linear accelerator radiosurgery or the gamma knife[®].

MR imaging, the most important imaging modality in SRS, requires special attention because it is well known that MR images show systemic geometric distortions which could limit their use in SRS. Image distortions and artefacts are present on all MR images. Artefacts are mostly patient related such as chemical shift or susceptibility artefacts and they change the local geometry of selected structures in the patient. These patient related artefacts are difficult to correct for and in principle limit geometric accuracy of MR images. In contrast, image distortions deriving from the MR scanner itself often affect all images within an imaging study. These systemic distortions, dependent on the imaging sequence applied, also limit localisation accuracy but can be measured by using dedicated phantoms. If necessary they can be corrected.

In Fig. 7a (upper figure) such a phantom is shown consisting of a water filled cylinder (17.5 cm in diameter and 13.4 cm in depth) and 145 embedded rods, 1 mm in diameter each, arranged on a regular grid with a grid constant of 10 mm. This phantom can precisely be mounted to the stereotactic frame, in order to place the middle rod exactly at the central stereotactic coordinate (x = y = 100 mm) in the central part of the image, where image distortion can usually be neglected. Together with the stereotactic MR localiser box the phantom is scanned using the identical imaging protocols as for patients undergoing SRS (see centre image Fig. 7a). The bottom image of Fig. 7 a shows a typical MR image of this phantom that can be analysed by dedicated software [15]. Figure 7b shows a screen shot of this analysis software which determines for each rod and each image the length of the displacement vector of the imaged rod position and its known actual rod position. Thus systemic image distortions can be detected. Not only different imaging protocols like 2D spin echo protocols or 3D volume acquisitions can be analysed in terms of image distortion but it is also possible to monitor changes occurring over a period of time due to changes in MR scanner components (head coil, shim and gradient coils).

Image distortions when using image intensifier based digital subtraction angiography (DSA) are also well known and are a source of uncertainty in the treatment chain. Because DSA images do not provide the three-dimensional structure of the lesion (typically AVMs), this imaging modality is often combined with CT and MR (MRA) imaging to overcome this limitation. In order to check the imaging accuracy of our image intensifier based DSA system, a grid phantom as shown in Fig. 8 top left is used, which consists of several 1 mm diameter steel spheres positioned on a 10 mm grid. On the top right side of Fig. 8 a typical image intensifier image of this phantom is shown where the typical "pin cushion" distortion can be noted towards the image edges. When a distortion free area in the central part of the image is assumed, the known marker position can be compared to the corresponding marker position found on the image. Figure 8 bottom left shows the radial dependence of the calculated length of the displacement vector for each marker found on the image. It can be seen that with increasing radius the displacement between known and detected position grows, reaching a maximum of over 3.5 mm. With the help of a dedicated correction algorithm this distortion can be corrected for and a subsequent analysis of the corrected image no longer shows such a systemic behaviour (Fig. 8 bottom right). Here the displacement vectors are less than 0.6 mm for all radii detected.

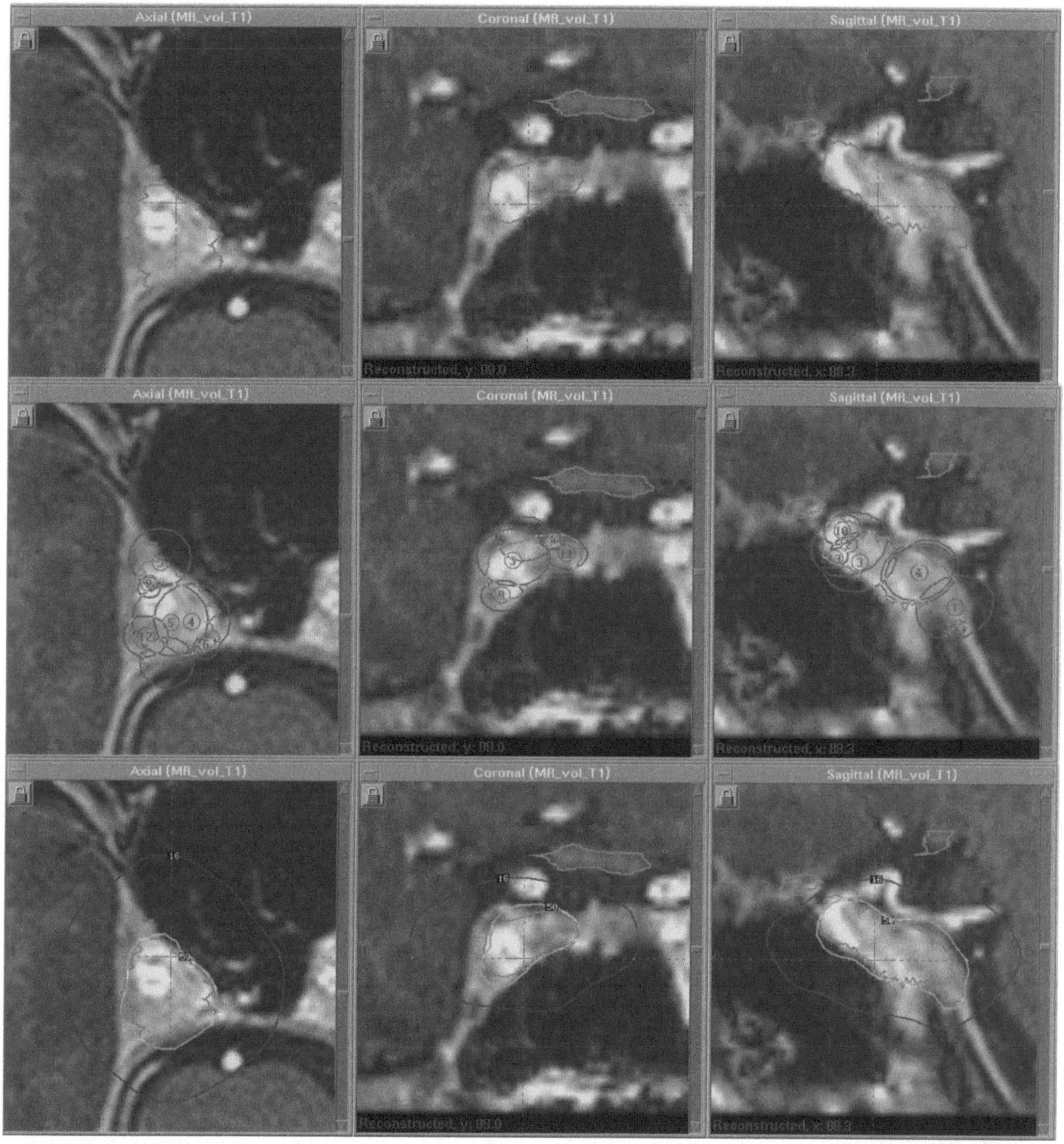

Fig. 4. Top row: Axial, coronal and sagittal views (from left to right) of T1 weighted MR images of the sella region showing a delineated pituitary adenoma (prolactinoma) together with the optic nerves as risk structures. The circles in the images of the middle row represent the different isocentre positions and sizes of the collimator helmets used to treat this lesion (5 × 8 mm and 8 × 4 mm collimator helmet) using multi-isocentric dose shaping. Bottom row: Resultant dose distribution in the axial, coronal and sagittal views. Note that the prescription isodose line (50% which corresponds in this case to 25 Gy) follows the target outline precisely and that the dose falls off very quickly, represented by the outer isodose line which represents 8 Gy in this case (16%)

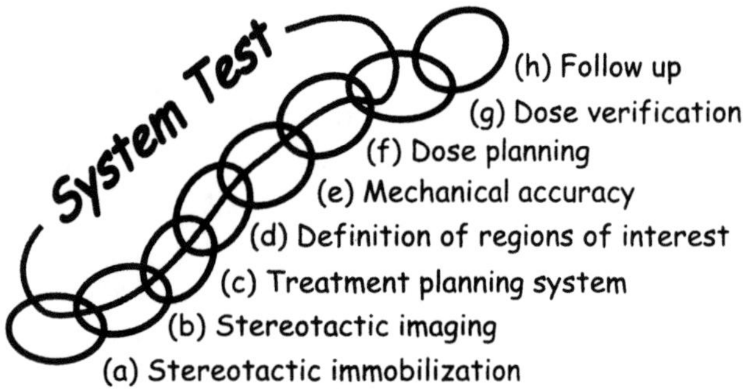

Fig. 5. The chain of uncertainties in radiosurgery. All technical uncertainties can be evaluated at the same time by use of the so-called "System Test"

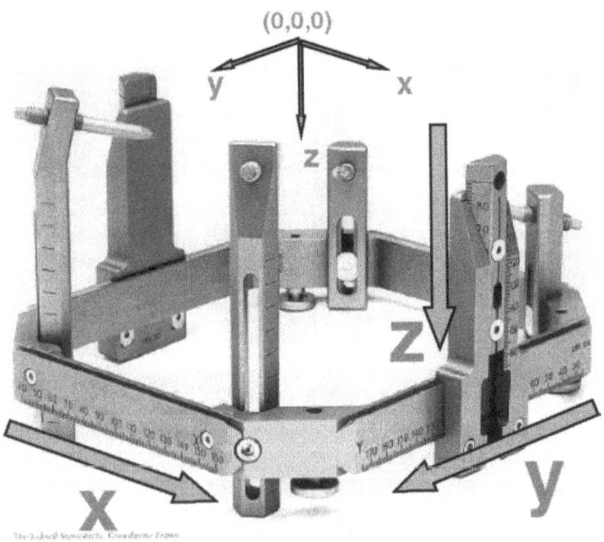

Fig. 6. The stereotactic Leksell frame used for immobilisation of the patient's skull defines a right handed Cartesian coordinate system with its origin at the right posterior top position

Treatment planning system

As a first step in treatment planning the stereotactic images – upon which treatment planning is based – have to be imported and stereotactically defined. This stereotactic image definition has to be checked in order to ensure a correct image orientation (left–right), correct image scaling and shear, as well as correct image resolution and spacing when calculating the elements of the rotation matrix based on the analyses of the known position of the fiducial markers in each image. With the help of this rotation matrix the stereotactic space is mapped to the stereotactic images. The accuracy of this procedure can be checked using the so-called "Known Target Point" method. In Fig. 9a a dedicated phantom is shown that can be used for CT and DSA imaging, mounted to the stereotactic frame together with the CT localiser box. The phantom consists of 8 lucite plates, in which altogether 45 steel spheres (diameter = 1 mm), positioned at known Leksell coordinates throughout the whole stereotactic space are embedded with a geometric accuracy of less than 0.1 mm. In figure 9b a single CT slice is shown where the known outer markers caused by the CT localiser box are used for stereotactic image definition. With the help of the treatment planning system, the stereotactic coordinates of the visible steel spheres can be determined and compared with their known true coordinates, resulting in a quantitative measure for the geometric image accuracy.

Definition of regions of interest (ROI)

As a next step in treatment planning the target and ROIs have to be determined based on several image modalities. For this an isotropic image resolution in 3d using small voxel sizes is adequate. When using multimodality imaging like DSA, CT, MRI, MRA, and PET, a detailed knowledge of the geometric accuracy of each image modality and possible image artefacts is necessary. Also clinical interpretation of different image modalities, which are operator dependent, has to be taken into account when defining ROIs.

Mechanical accuracy

In contrast to the links of the chain described so far, measuring the mechanical accuracy of a treatment unit is different for each irradiation technique used, although the basic principle is quite comparable. Illustrated here is the procedure for the gamma knife®. In order to check how well the UCP corresponds with the radiologic centre, which is the centroid of the superimposed dose distribution of all 201 beams, a special tool is provided by the manufacturer. In Fig. 10 a this tool is shown; the UCP is indicated by the tip of a needle. A radiochromic film is sandwiched with this tool, pierced by the needle and then irradiated. As schematically indicated in Fig. 10 b the centroid of the resultant dose distribution could be off centre with respect to UCP if the beam axes are not perfectly aligned. In this case the centroid of dose distribution as shown in Fig. 10 c in two of the three directions does not correspond with the position of the needle tip, which is indicated by the dip in the dose profile shown in Fig. 10 d. Through appropriate orientation of the special tool together with the film, the distance of the radiological centre from the UCP can be determined for each axis. The mean value of our measurements in Zurich for the mean radial deviation is 0.159 mm. For comparison: the mechanical accuracy of linear accelerator based units is usually greater than 1.0 mm [20] and about 0.5 to 0.9 mm using an additional floor stand [5].

Dose planning

Quality assurance in dose planning is highly operator dependent. In theory we aim for full dose within the target and zero dose outside. Because this is physically not achievable, we try to maximise the dose to the target and to minimise the dose outside. In SRS with gamma knife® this can be achieved by using a sufficient number of smaller collimator sizes. With the help of an automatic positioning system (APS) available for gamma knife® C, an increased number of shots can be applied without spending too much time on manually repositioning the patient. Figure 11 gives a clear impression of the improvement regarding dose shaping when comparing a dose distribution (50% isodose line) based on a larger single shot (axial, coronal and sagittal view, upper row) with a corresponding multi-shot dose plan using 15 smaller shots (bottom row in figure 11). From Fig. 11 it can also be seen that the higher isodose lines (75% in this example) encompass a larger portion of the target when only a low number of shots is used. This potential benefit in terms of lesion control is counterbalanced by a significantly higher probability of complication in the surrounding healthy tissue, which in this case receives a significantly higher dose. This statement leads to the more general

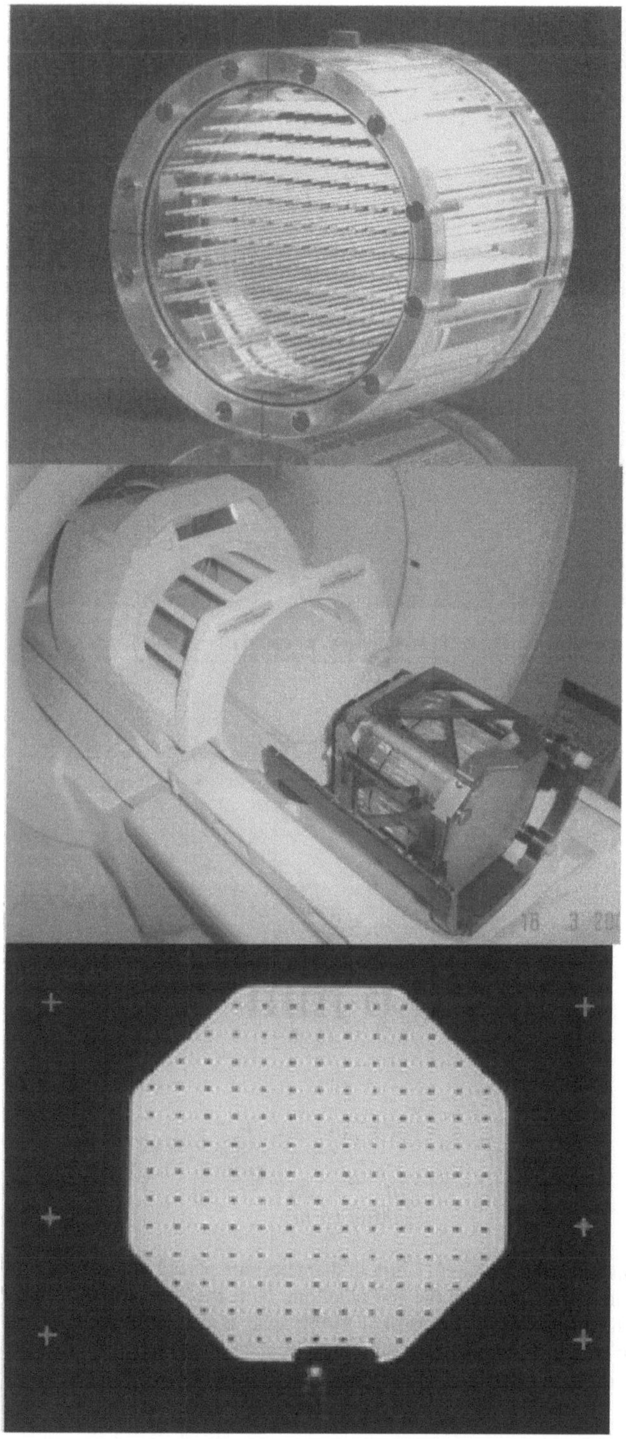

a

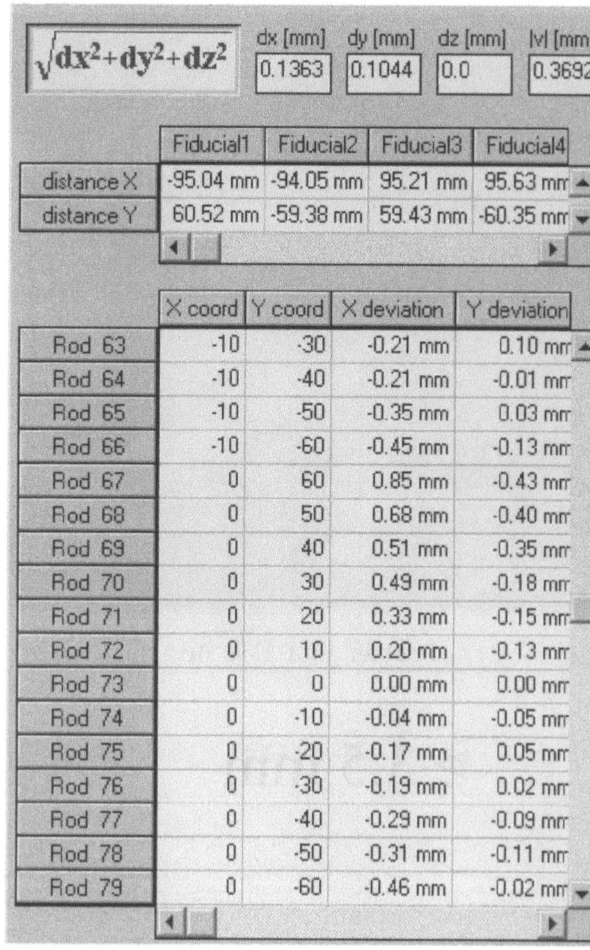

$\sqrt{dx^2+dy^2+dz^2}$	dx [mm]	dy [mm]	dz [mm]	lvl [mm]
	0.1363	0.1044	0.0	0.3692

	Fiducial1	Fiducial2	Fiducial3	Fiducial4
distance X	-95.04 mm	-94.05 mm	95.21 mm	95.63 mm
distance Y	60.52 mm	-59.38 mm	59.43 mm	-60.35 mm

	X coord	Y coord	X deviation	Y deviation
Rod 63	-10	-30	-0.21 mm	0.10 mm
Rod 64	-10	-40	-0.21 mm	-0.01 mm
Rod 65	-10	-50	-0.35 mm	0.03 mm
Rod 66	-10	-60	-0.45 mm	-0.13 mm
Rod 67	0	60	0.85 mm	-0.43 mm
Rod 68	0	50	0.68 mm	-0.40 mm
Rod 69	0	40	0.51 mm	-0.35 mm
Rod 70	0	30	0.49 mm	-0.18 mm
Rod 71	0	20	0.33 mm	-0.15 mm
Rod 72	0	10	0.20 mm	-0.13 mm
Rod 73	0	0	0.00 mm	0.00 mm
Rod 74	0	-10	-0.04 mm	-0.05 mm
Rod 75	0	-20	-0.17 mm	0.05 mm
Rod 76	0	-30	-0.19 mm	0.02 mm
Rod 77	0	-40	-0.29 mm	-0.09 mm
Rod 78	0	-50	-0.31 mm	-0.11 mm
Rod 79	0	-60	-0.46 mm	-0.02 mm

b

Fig. 7. (a) Photograph of the water filled cylindrical phantom with 145 embedded rods. The rods are positioned equidistantly in a 10 mm grid (top). The middle photograph shows the cylindrical rod phantom, mounted in the stereotactic Leksell frame together with the localiser box prepared for MR-scanning. The bottom image shows the corresponding axial MR image where the position of the rods can be clearly seen. (b) Screen shot of the analysis software which is used to analyse MR images by comparing the known rod position within the stereotactic space with the corresponding position found in the MR image. For each rod the calculated deviation in x and y is shown and indicates a displacement vector due to image distortions

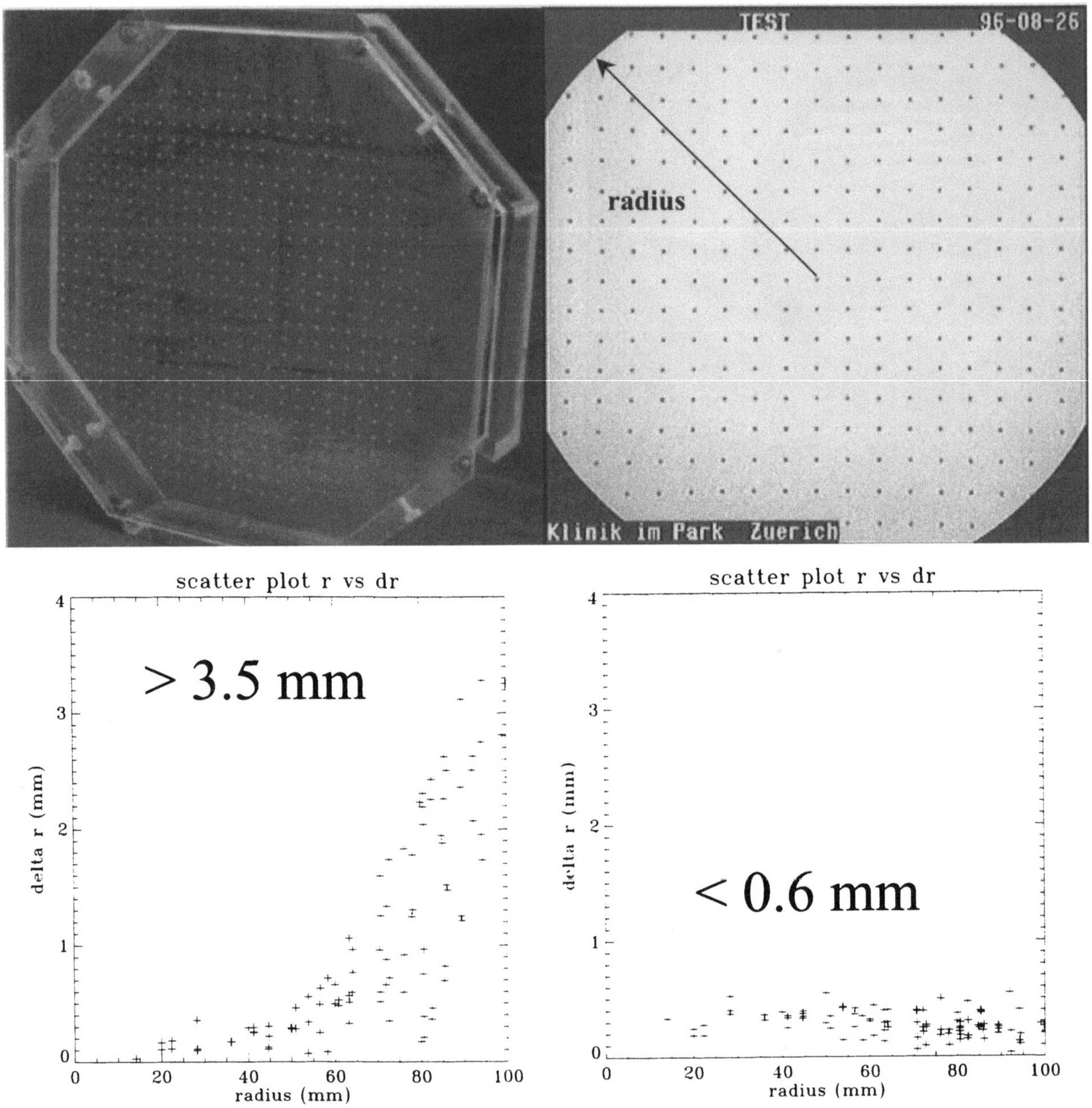

Fig. 8. Top left: Grid phantom used for image intensifier based DSA imaging. Steel spheres (1 mm in diameter) are placed in a regular grid (grid distance = 10 mm) within a Lucite plate. Top right: Typical image intensifier image of the grid phantom. Note the "pin cushion" image distortion at peripheral regions of the image. Bottom left: The length of the displacement vectors of all visible spheres are plotted against their radial distance from the central marker. Note the increasing displacement with increasing radius. Bottom right: After applying an appropriate image distortion correction algorithm, the radial dependence of the image distortion can be corrected. After correction all markers in the image were found to be within 0.6 mm of their geometric position

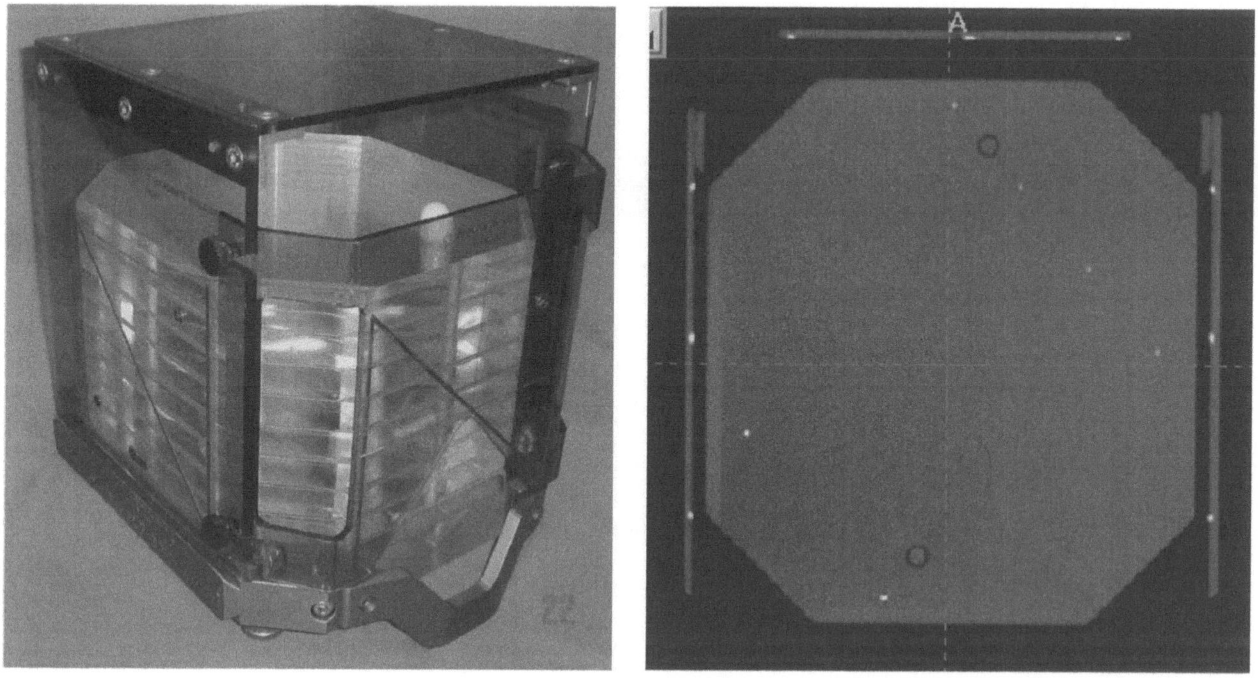

a b

Fig. 9. (a) Photograph of the CT (and DSA) phantom consisting of 8 lucite plates, containing 45 steel spheres (1 mm in diameter), distributed throughout the stereotactic space at known Leksell coordinates, mounted in the stereotactic frame together with the CT localiser box. (b) Axial CT image of the phantom with several steel spheres and fiducial markers visible. By comparing the stereotactic coordinates of the embedded marker after stereotactic coordinate definition using the treatment planning system with the known coordinates, the geometric accuracy of the CT images and the stereotactic coordinate transformation can be checked

question of how to score the different dose plans for a patient, or how to decide on the treatment modality to offer superior dose distributions when comparing different technical implementations for SRS [11]. In contrast to dose plans applied with the gamma knife®, where prescription dose is often defined at the 50% isodose, the 80% isodose is typically chosen in a linear accelerator based treatment. This difference in percentage prescription dose increases the mean dose to the target when using the gamma knife®, assuming the same prescription dose is given for both treatment techniques.

Dose verification

Dose verifications are necessary to check the congruence of the calculated and the measured dose distributions [10]. A first quantity that has to be measured for all treatment units is the so-called output factor. For the gamma knife® the absolute dose rate is measured only for the largest, the 18 mm collimator helmet, with a calibrated air ionisation chamber. For this helmet the dose distribution shows a relatively large plateau region as seen in Fig. 3. The dose rates for the smaller collimator helmets are then calculated by multiplying the dose rate measured for the 18 mm collimator with the corresponding output factor of the smaller ones. The output factor for the 18 mm collimator per definition is 1.0. The output factors decrease with decreasing beam diameter and can be measured using relative dosimetry methods and dedicated detectors. Details have been described in the paper by Mack and Scheib *et al.* [17]. The respective measured dose profiles for the gamma knife® are shown in figure 3 and have to be compared to the calculated profiles using the treatment planning system. In order to verify dose distributions in a more realistic way dedicated phantoms have to be used which are handled in the same manner as a real patient. Figure 12 shows a dose verification experiment using an anthropomorphic phantom and radiochromic film [12, 14, 24]. The experiment assumed a CPA schwannoma in the phantom which was irradiated with seven 8 mm and four 4 mm shots. The right side of Fig. 12 shows the percentage isodose lines of the measured dose distribution. By applying an appropriate calibration curve absolute 2D distributions can also be measured with this method. For direct 3D dose measurements one has to stack either several radiochromic films or use dosimetry gels which are 3D dosimeters. In Fig. 13 an example of a measured relative dose distribution (broken isodose lines), compared to the calculated dose distribution (solid isodose lines) is shown in an axial, coronal and sagittal view together with the corresponding relative dose images based on R_2 measurement which is proportional to the absorbed dose [25].

Follow up

As an important parameter to assess the efficacy of a treatment, each patient has to undergo several clinical follow-up examinations. At our site, most of the patients receive their image based follow-up study in our neuroradiological department, facilitating image data transfer based on the dicom standard. In order to follow volumetric changes of the treated lesion, a dedicated software has been developed in-house [23] by means of which the volume of structures out-

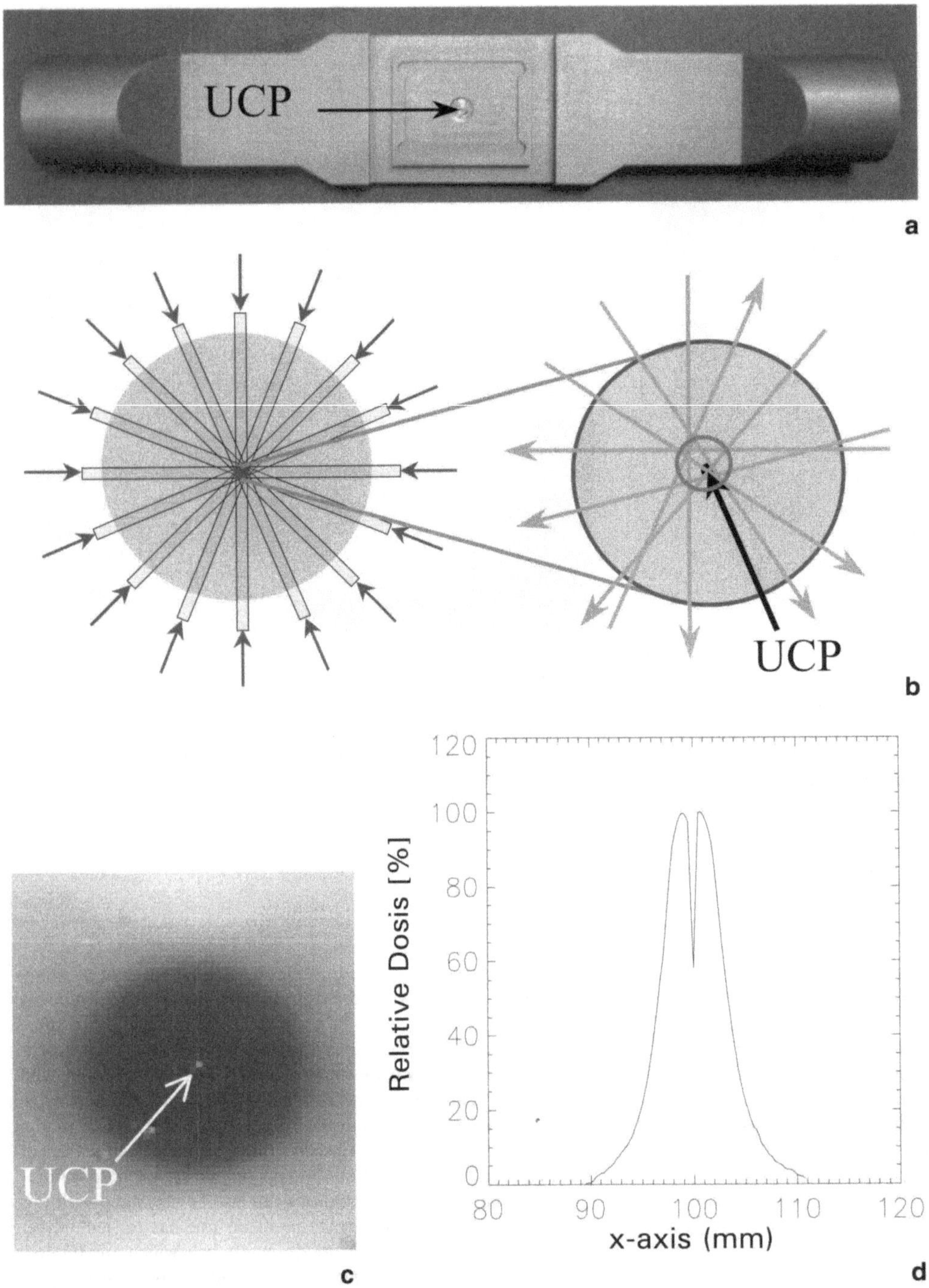

Fig. 10. (a) Special tool provided together with the gamma knife® to check the deviation between the mechanical isocentre (Unit Centre Point – UCP) represented by the needle tip and the radiological isocentre, which is the centre of the superimposed dose distribution of all single beams. For this measurement a radiochromic film is positioned in the special tool and pierced by the tip of the needle prior to irradiation. (b) Schematic representation of the cross firing 201 beams in the gamma knife® (left). The UCP region (zoomed area on the right) is shown together with the geometric (mechanical) centre indicated by the arrow head and the centre of the beam axes (centre of the inner circle) which do not necessarily coincide. (c) A pierced radiochromic film is irradiated with the help of the special tool and analysed in order to determine the deviation of the radiological isocentre (centre of the dose distribution) and the mechanical (*UCP*) isocentre along all three stereotactic axes. (d) Dose profile along the x-axis used to calculate the deviation in x by analysing the radiological centre based on the full width at half maximum (*FWHM*) and the dip in the dose distribution caused by the piercing

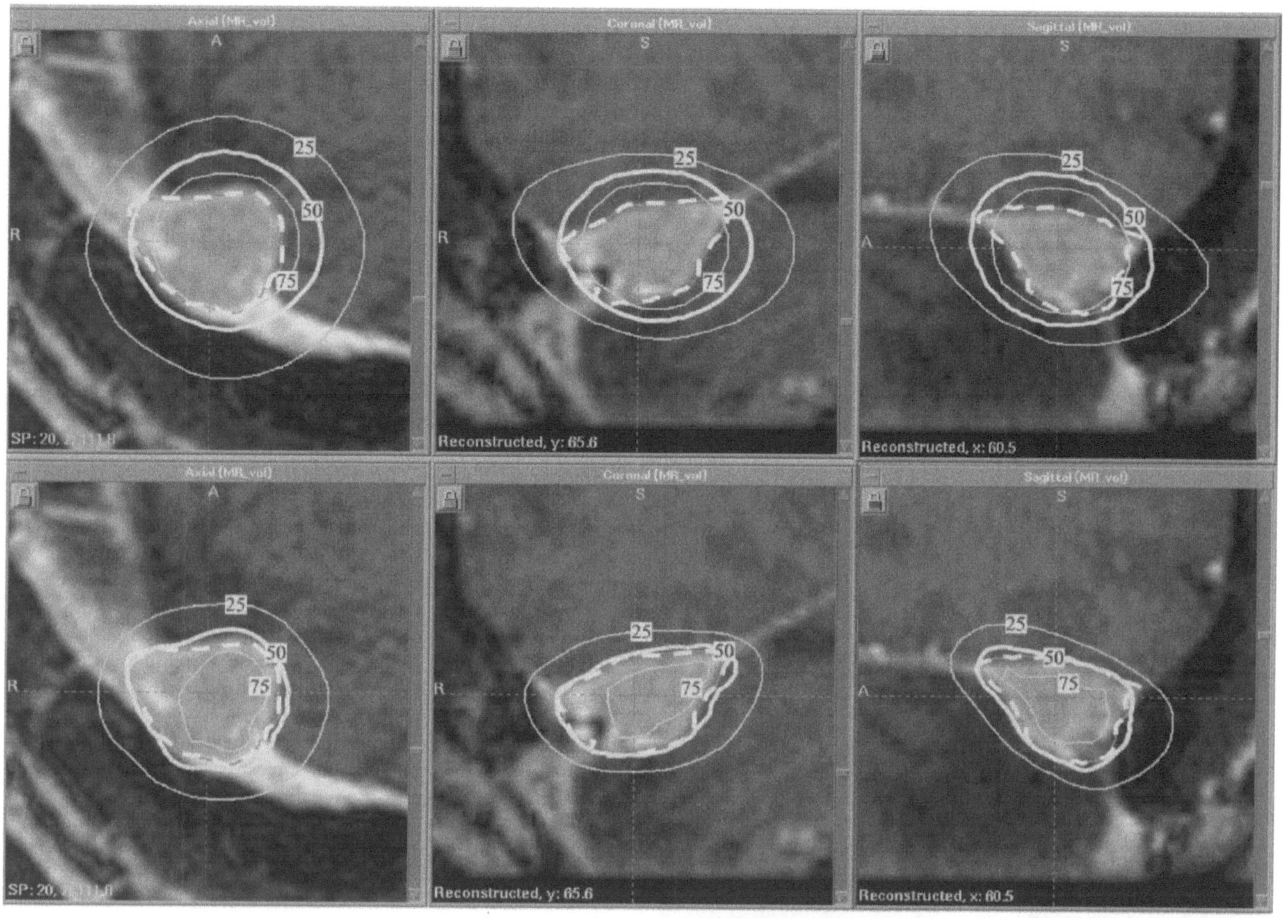

Fig. 11. Axial, coronal and sagittal (from left to right) view of a dose plan for a meningioma (target volume = 1.4 cm^3) in the region of the right transverse sinus using a larger single shot (top row) compared to a conformal multishot (multi-isocentric) plan using 15 smaller shots

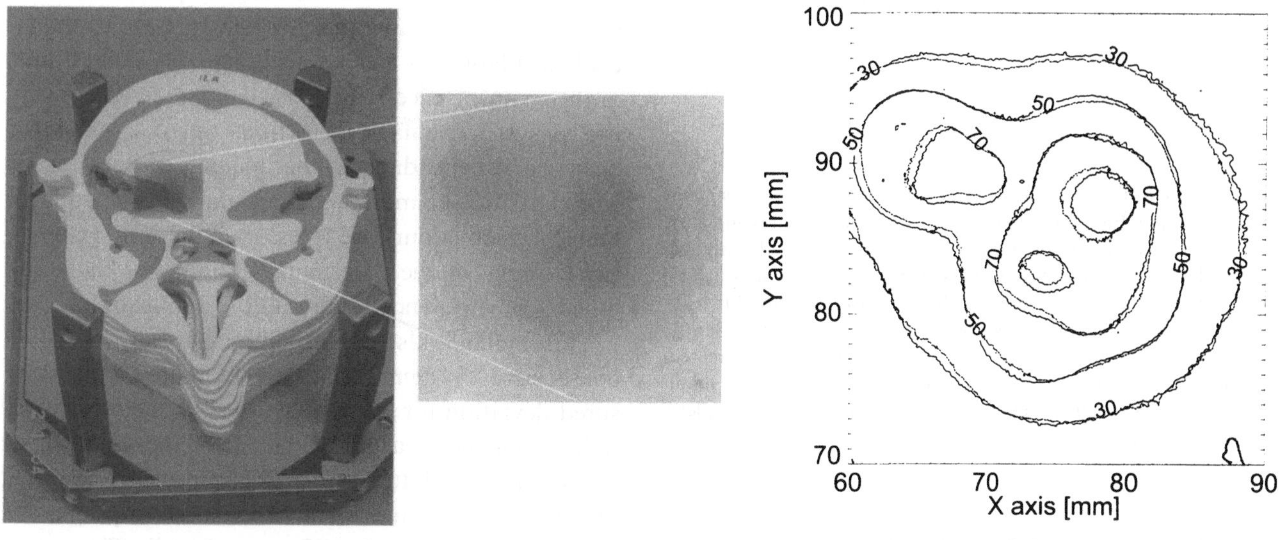

Fig. 12. Lower part of a dismantled anthropomorphic head phantom (left) shown together with a radiochromic film (middle) after application of a multi-isocentric treatment (7 × 8 mm and 4 × 4 mm collimator helmet) for a simulated CPA schwannoma. By applying an appropriate calibration curve to the radiochromic film, measured isodose lines can be extracted (right) and compared to calculated ones

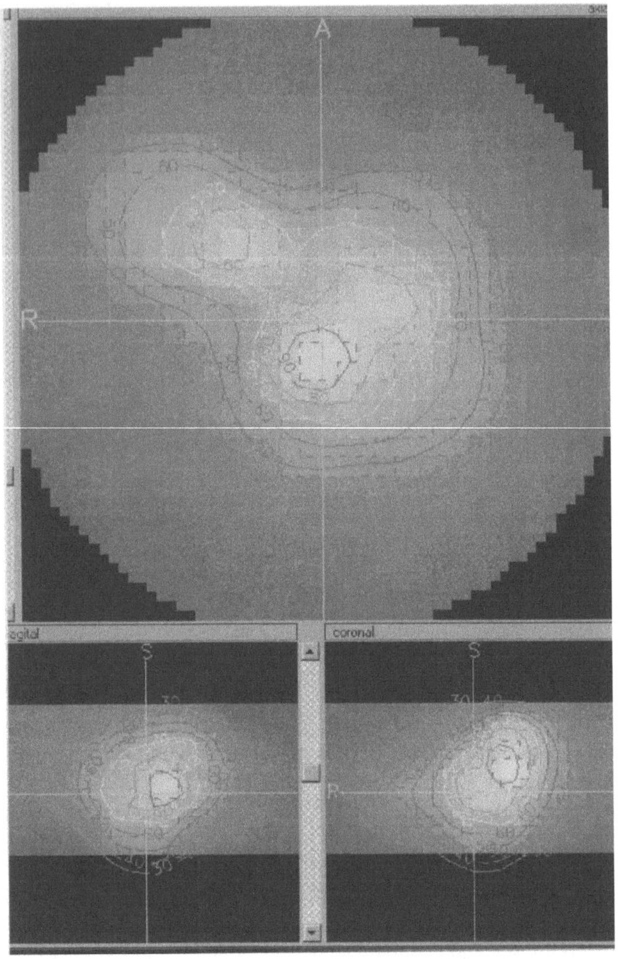

Fig. 13. Axial (top), sagittal (bottom left) and coronal (bottom right) view of calculated (solid lines) and measured (broken lines) isodose lines (30, 40, 50, 60, 80 and 90%) together with the relative dose image for a typical multi-isocentric CPA schwannoma treatment using BANG^{TM}-25 gel and the anthropomorphic phantom shown in Fig. 12

lined on MR or CT slices are determined without need for a stereotactic definition. Figure 14 shows a typical volumetric follow-up over a period of five years for a CPA schwannoma treated with the gamma knife®. As line measurements are not sufficiently sensitive to small volume changes, we prefer volume measurements. This is illustrated in figure 15 showing a graphic representation of the lesion volume measured with this software. The graph shows an increased lesion volume of about 20% one year after treatment, which cannot be attributed to a treatment failure considering the subsequent follow-up studies.

System test

By performing a stereotactic irradiation using a spherical phantom and radiochromic film, handled like a real patient, the accuracy of the whole chain of uncertainties including immobilisation, stereotactic imaging, dose calculation, irradiation and set-up of phantom in the treatment unit is simultaneously checked by delivering a single isocentre irradiation (4 mm collimator). In Fig. 15 the workflow of this system test is illustrated, starting with a visible target point using diagnostic imaging modalities (cross-over point of the cross hair filled with copper sulphate solution), placed within the spherical phantom, through to a software assisted analysis of the irradiated radiochromic film which is marked with several dots for correct orientation and a premarked cross placed over the cross-over point of the cross hair prior to starting the procedure [15].

Technical standards

The aim of technical standards is to define key terms in the field of SRS, to outline test methods for commissioning and functional performance tests, to determine levels of accuracy and precision for different technical implementations for radiosurgery and to recommend time intervals for the described tests. Over the last decade several contributions concerning quality assurance and technical standards have been published. In the book edited by M. Phillips [19] some acceptance tests for SRS implementations are described. A more detailed collection of acceptance and regular constancy checks is contained in the booklet edited by G. Hartmann [8] and the report on stereotactic radiosurgery published by a task group upon initiation by the American Association of Physicists in Medicine (AAPM) [27]. In addition to these reports, the international electrotechnical commission (IEC) (technical committee no 62, electrical equipment in medical practice) has also published a report focusing on particular safety requirements [9]. The most recent technical standards have been issued by DIN under the supervision of the "Normenausschuss Radiologie" and are entitled: "DIN 6875-1: Special radiotherapy equipments – Part 1: Percutaneous stereotactic radiotherapy, basic performance characteristics and essential test methods" [4].

Results

The quality assurance tests described are mostly independent of the treatment unit used for radiosurgery and are compatible with the recently published DIN 6875-1. Phantoms and analyses software are commercially available. As regards accuracy, the weakest link in the chain of uncertainties is stereotactic MR imaging as systemic image distortions up to 2 mm have been found depending on the imaging protocol used. Compared to the mechanical accuracy of the gamma knife®, which in our case is less than 0.2 mm, geometric accuracy of the MR images dominates the combined geometric uncertainty of dose application.

This finding is also confirmed by the analyses of 170 consecutive "System Tests" [15]. In figure 16 the measured deviation for each system test of the cross-over point from the measured centroid of the 4 mm dose distribution is plotted for a 2D spin echo sequence (filled diamonds) and for a 3D volume (mprage) sequence as used for the "System Tests". The mean value using the 2D spin echo sequence is 0.66 mm and 0.4 mm using the 3D volume sequence. It has also

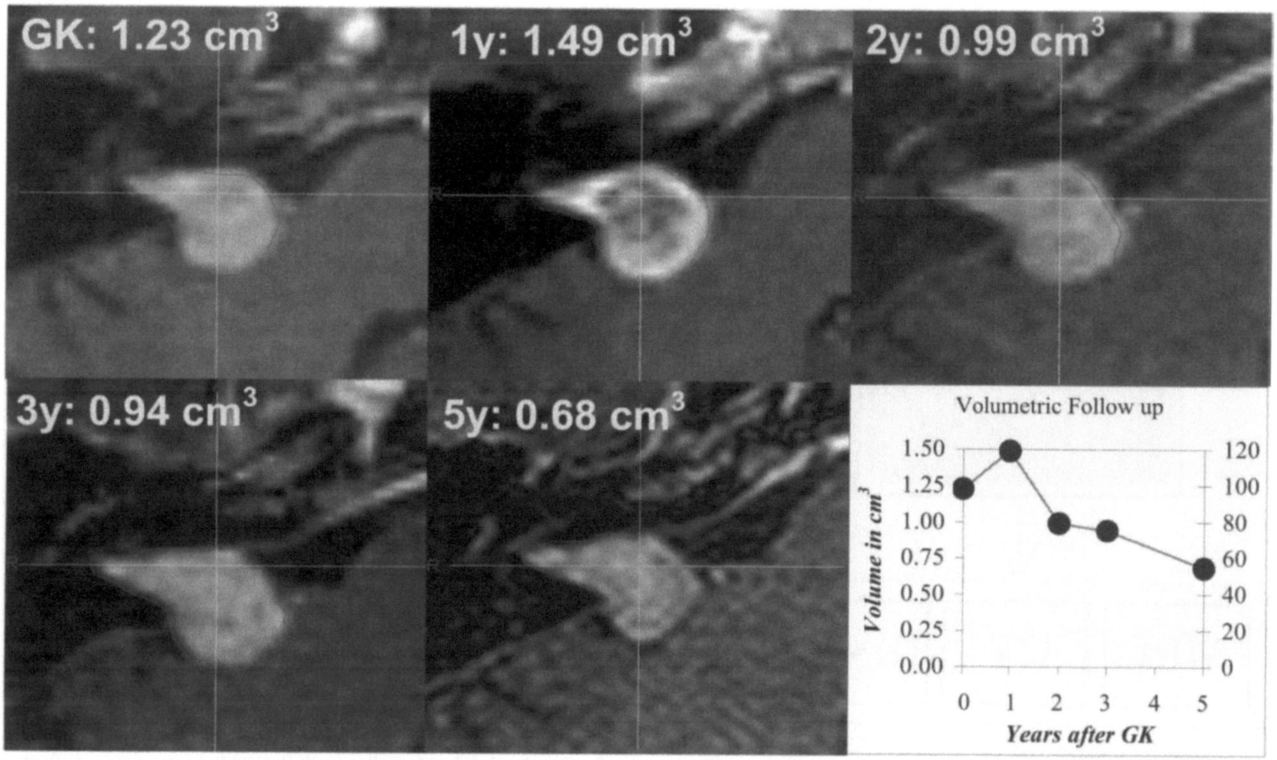

Fig. 14. Typical volumetric follow-up study for a CPA schwannoma treated with the gamma knife® covering a follow-up period of 5 years. Note the transient volume increase in the follow-up image one year after treatment

been found that it cannot in general be stated that 3D volume acquisition protocols in MR imaging are superior to 2D imaging protocols in terms of geometric accuracy. For each MR scanner and magnetic field strength the imaging sequences under consideration have to be evaluated in order to check their geometric accuracy.

Discussion

Given the high mechanical accuracy and stability of the Leksell Gamma Knife®, the most sensitive technical factor having an influence on overall accuracy in radiosurgery is MR imaging. Detailed analyses of all links in the chain of uncertainties guarantee a geometric and dosimetric accuracy of treatment which is well within clinically based and standardised tolerances. Apart from imaging this accuracy will unlikely change on a day-to-day basis and can be monitored using available and clinically validated tools for routine quality assurance which are in agreement with published technical standards.

Besides the possibility to apply highly conformal, three dimensional dose distributions accurately to selected structures there is still potential for improvements in gamma knife® based radiosurgery taking into account the growing interest in neuroscience. Further improvements should focus on geometric imaging accuracy still dominating overall accuracy. Also further refinements in the quality assurance procedures described are useful to speed up test procedures. Furthermore the potential of dynamic in focus positioning of the patient within the gamma knife® together with optimised dose distributions is under discussion. When compared to other clinical implementations in SRS, the gamma knife® has become a standard by itself.

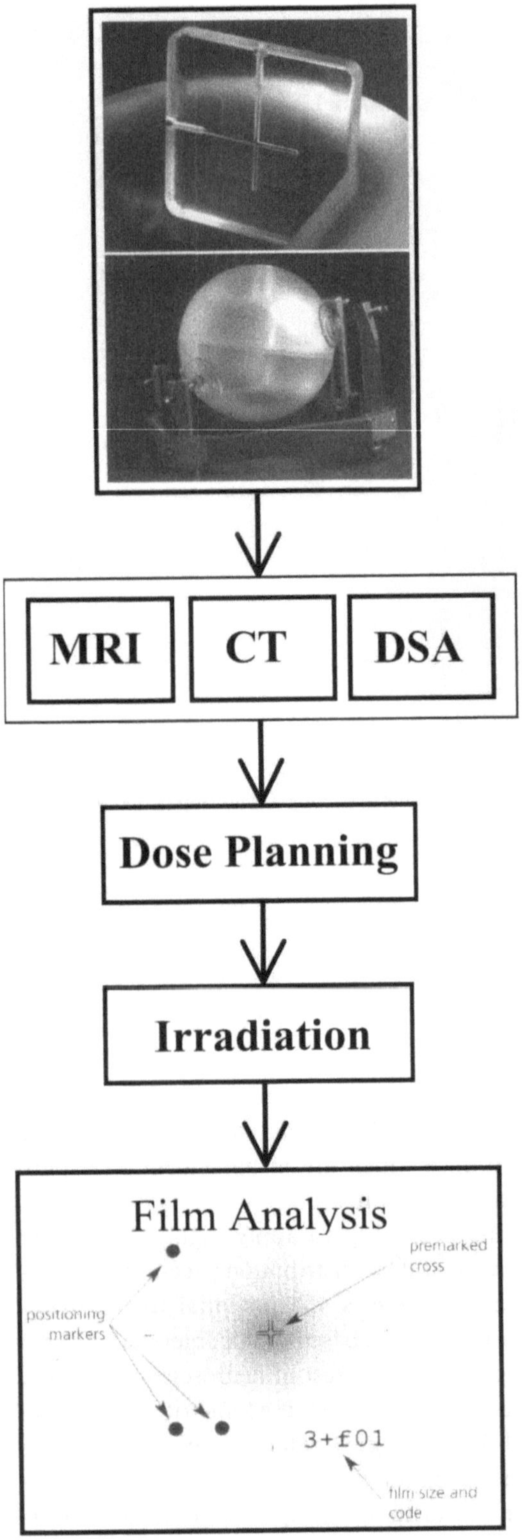

Fig. 15. Workflow of the system test checking the chain of uncertainties (see Fig. 5)

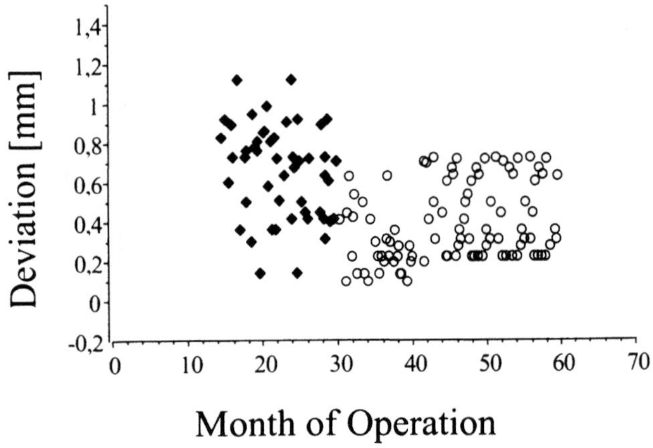

Fig. 16. Results of 170 consecutive system tests using 2D Spin Echo (SE) MR imaging (filled diamonds) and 3D (mprage) MR imaging (open circles). The mean value is 0.66 mm for 2D SE and 0.4 mm for 3D MR imaging

References

1. Alexander III E, Loeffler JS, Lunsford LD (1993) Stereotactic radiosurgery. McGraw-Hill
2. Bourland JD, McCollough KP (1994) Static field conformal stereotactic radiosurgery: physical techniques. Int J Radiat Oncol Biol Phys 28: 471–479
3. Cardinale RM, Benedict SH, Wu Q, Zwicker RD, Gaballa HE, Mohan R (1998) A comparison of three stereotactic radiotherapy techniques: ARCS vs. noncoplanar fixed fields vs. intensity modulation. Int J Radiat Oncol Biol Phys 42: 431–436
4. DIN 6875-1 (2004) Spezielle Bestrahlungseinrichtungen – Teil 1: Perkutane stereotaktische Bestrahlung, Kennmerkmale und besondere Prüfmethoden. Normenausschuss Radiologie (NAR) im DIN Deutsches Institut für Normung e.V., Beuth Verlag, Berlin
5. Engler MJ, Curran BH, Tsai JS, Sternick ES, Selles WD, Wazer DE, Mason WP, Sailor T, Mackie TR (1994) Fine tuning of linear accelerator accessories for stereotactic radiotherapy. Int J Radiat Oncol Biol Phys 28: 1001–1008
6. Ertl A, Saringer W, Heimberger K, Kindl P (1999) Quality assurance for the Leksell gamma unit: considering magnetic resonance image-distortion and delineation failure in the targeting of the internal auditory canal. Med Phys 26: 166–170
7. Friedman WA, Buatti JM, Bova FJ, Mendenhall WM (1997) Linac radiosurgery – a practical guide. Springer, Berlin Heidelberg New York Tokyo
8. Hartmann GH (1995) Quality assurance program on stereotactic radiosurgery. Springer, Berlin Heidelberg New York Tokyo
9. IEC 60601-2-11 (1997) Medical electrical equipment – part 2: particular requirements for the safety of gamma beam therapy equipment. International Electrotechnical Commission, Technical Committee No 62, Electrical Equipment in medical practice
10. Jess A, Kreiner HJ, Heck B, Wowra B, Mack A (2003) Bestrahlungsplanung bei kleinen complex geformten Läsionen und ihre experimentelle Verifikation. Z Med Phys 13: 16–21
11. Lomax NJ, Scheib SG (2003) Quantifying the degree of conformity in radiosurgery treatment planning. Int J Radiat Oncol Biol Phys 55: 1409–1419

12. Mack A, Mack G, Weltz D, Scheib S, Böttcher H, Seifert V (2003) High precision film dosimetry with GAFCHROMIC® films for quality assurance when using small fields. Med Phys 30: 2399–2409
13. Mack A, Mack G, Weltz D, Hönes A, Jess A, Wowra B, Czempiel H, Heck B, Kreiner HJ, Seifert V, Böttcher H (2003) Qualitätssicherung im stereotaktischen Raum. Bestimmung der Genauigkeit von Ort und Dosis bei Einzeit-Bestrahlungen. Strahlentherapie und Onkologie 179: 760–766
14. Mack A (2002) Verification of dose plans using film dosimetry for quality assurance in radiosurgery. In: Kondziolka D (ed) Radiosurgery. Karger, Basel, vol 4, pp 213–227
15. Mack A, Czempiel H, Kreiner HJ, Dürr G, Wowra B (2002) Quality assurance in stereotactic space, a system test for verifying the accuracy of aim in radiosurgery. Med Phys 29: 561–568
16. Mack A, Weltz D, Czempiel H, Beck B, Kreiner HJ, Wolff R, Mack G (2002) Experimentally determined 3-d dose distributions of small, complex targets. J Neurosurg [Suppl] 5(97): 551–555
17. Mack A, Scheib SG, Major J, Gianolini S, Pazmandi G, Feist H, Czempiel H, Kreiner HJ (2002) Precision dosimetry for narrow photon beams used in radiosurgery – determination of gamma knife output factors. Med Phys 29: 2080–2089
18. Maitz AH, Wu A, Lunsford LD, Flickinger JC, Kondziolka D, Bloomer WD (1995) Quality assurance for gamma knife stereotactic radiosurgery. Int J Radiat Oncol Biol Phys 32: 1465–1471
19. Phillips MH (1993) Physical aspects of stereotactic radiosurgery. Plenum Medical Book Company, New York London
20. Ramaseshan R, Heydarian M (2003) Comprehensive quality assurance for stereotactic radiosurgery treatments. Phys Med Biol 48: N199–205
21. Rosenzweig DP, Schell MC, Numaguchi Y (1998) Quality assurance in linac-based stereotactic radiosurgery and radiotherapy. Med Dosim 23: 147–151
22. Schad LR, Ehricke HH, Wowra B *et al* (1992) Correction of spatial distortion in magnetic resonance angiography for radiosurgical treatment planning of cerebral arteriovenous malformations. Magn Reson Imaging 10: 609–621
23. Scheib SG, Gianolini S, Haller D, Wellis GN, Siegried J (2000) VOLUMESERIES: a software tool for target volume follow-up studies with computerized tomography and magnetic resonance imaging. J Neurosurg [Suppl] 3(93): 203–207
24. Scheib SG, Gianolini S (2002) Methodology of three-dimensional dosimetric dose verification in radiosurgery. In: Kondziolka D (ed) Radiosurgery. Karger, Basel, vol 4, pp 203–212
25. Scheib SG, Gianolini S (2002) Three-dimensional dose verification using BANG gel: a clinical example. J Neurosurg [Suppl] 5(97): 582–587
26. Scheib SG, Mack A, Lomax NJ, Gianolini S, Hönes A, Rieker M, Weltz D (2003) Quality assurance in stereotactic radiosurgery according E-DIN 6875-1. Proceedings of the joint meeting of the Swiss Society of Radiation Biology and Medical Physics and the Scientific Association of Swiss Radiation Oncology, Geneva, April 3–5
27. Schell MC, Bova FJ, Larson DA, Leavitt DD, Lutz WR, Podgorsak, Wu A (1995) AAPM Report No. 54. Stereotactic radiosurgery. Report of Task Group 42. American Institute of Physics, New York, NY
28. Wowra B, Czempiel H, Cibis R, Horstmann GA (1997) Profil der ambulanten Radiochirurgie mit dem Gamma-Knife-System, Teil 1: Methode und multizentrisches Bestrahlungskonzept. Radiologe 37: 995–1002

Correspondence: Stefan G. Scheib, Ph.D., Department of Medical Radiation Physics, Klinik Im Park, Seestrasse 220, 8027 Zurich, Switzerland. e-mail: stefan.scheib@hirslanden.ch

Acta Neurochir (2004) [Suppl] 91: 25–32

Clinical quality standards for gamma knife radiosurgery – The Munich protocol –

A. Muacevic[1], **A. Jess-Hempen**[1], **J.-C. Tonn**[2], and **B. Wowra**[1]

[1] German Gamma Knife Center Munich, Ludwig-Maximilians University Munich, Munich, Germany
[2] Department of Neurosurgery, Ludwig-Maximilians University Munich, Munich, Germany

Summary

The clinical quality standards for outpatient gamma knife radiosurgery as developed in the German Gamma Knife Center Munich during the last ten years are described. The following aspects have been taken into account: appropriate patient selection, standardised treatment cycle, acquisition of high-quality stereotactic MR images, the integrated therapeutic concept, dose conformity and dose level, patient follow-up, quality control and scientific data analysis. Particular emphasis has been put on the importance of the interdisciplinary treatment concept by subspecialised experts. The results of the Munich concept in consideration of the described quality standards verifies that gamma knife radiosurgery is a safe and effective treatment option for well selected indications.

Keywords: Gamma knife; radiosurgery; quality standards; interdisciplinary treatment concept.

Gamma knife radiosurgery quality standards

Gamma knife radiosurgery must incorporate rigid quality standards, given the goal of delivering a high single dose of radiation to small intracranial tissue volumes with the participation of multiple disciplines. The current configuration of the device is considered to be the gold standard treatment platform for stereotactic radiosurgery within the brain [5, 11]. The gamma knife is a dedicated unit which is ideally refined for its single purpose. It is considered the most accurate device for radiosurgery and it combines high precision irradiations and a steep dose gradient to minimize the dose to the surrounding tissue. It is clinically effective in treating certain benign and malignant brain tumours, arteriovenous malformations, trigeminal neuralgia and other more rare indications. 3000 patients have been treated by outpatient radiosurgery in Munich, Germany from October 1994 to September 2004. To guarantee a high quality standard, a comprehensive clinical and technical quality assurance program is essential. Highest precision can only be achieved when all potential mechanical/technical errors and all clinical errors are reduced to a minimum. The following clinical quality parameters are regarded as essential for a successful radiosurgical treatment:

- appropriate patient selection
- standardized treatment cycle
- acquisition of high-quality, distortion-free 3-D stereotactic MR images
- integrated therapeutic concept
- high dose conformity
- appropriate dose level
- specific clinical and radiographical patient follow-up
- quality control – monitoring complications
- scientific data analysis

All of these elements are critical, and poor performance of any part will lead to suboptimal results. This chapter deals with the clinical quality standards developed in the German Gamma Knife Center Munich during the past 10 years. The above mentioned elements will be discussed in this chapter.

Appropriate patient selection

The evolution in patient selection together with better imaging and computer work stations have led to improved results. Standard indications for gamma knife radiosurgery are arteriovenous malformations, benign tumors (meningiomas, acoustic neurinomas), malignant tumors (metastases), and trigeminal neuralgia (Fig. 1). The therapeutic impact of each tumor entity is discussed in the specific chapters of this book. To select the correct patient for a gamma knife proce-

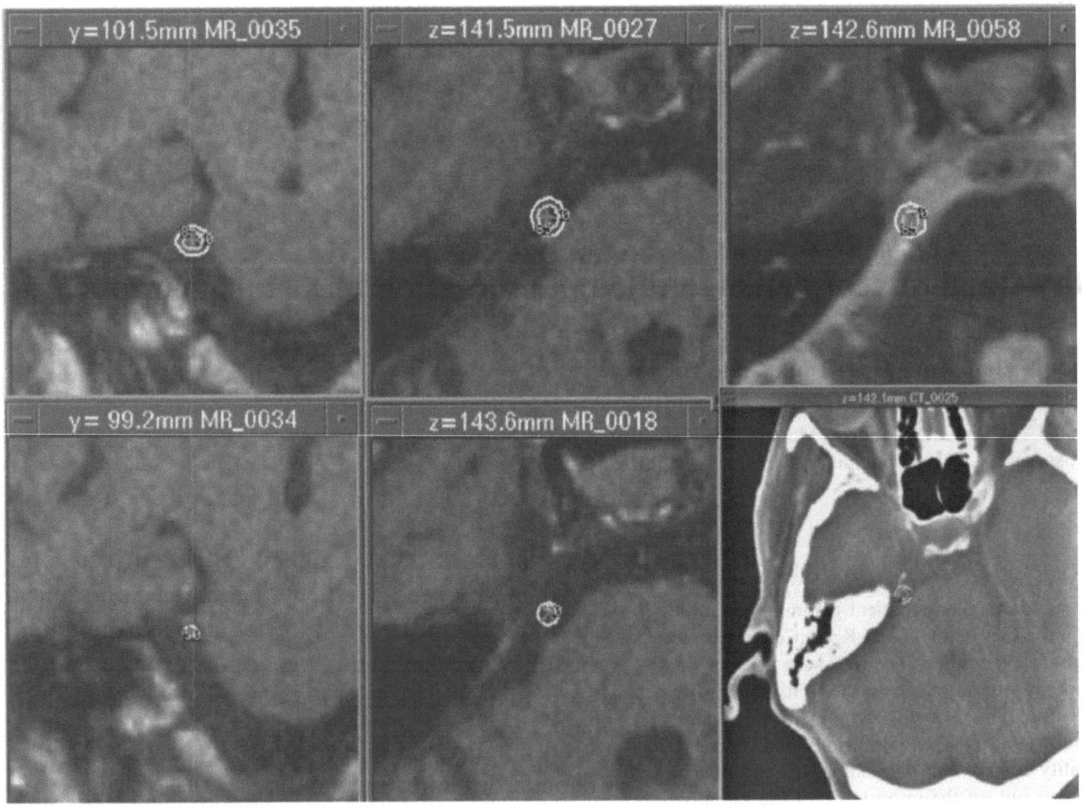

Fig. 1. Shows an example for gamma knife treatment planning in a patient suffering from persistent right sided trigeminal neuralgia after microvascular decompression. The coronal and axial MRI plan demonstrates the demand for highest accuracy in selected cases. The target has a diameter of about 3 mm. In the right lower corner the corresponding CT scan is shown

dure can be a difficult task. It is therefore of utmost importance that the responsible radiosurgeon be a fully trained neurosurgeon. Otherwise it is not possible to thoroughly explore the potential risks and benefits for gamma knife surgery in each individual case. This is particularly true for skull base tumors like acoustic neuromas and meningiomas where the involvement of cranial nerves and important vascular structures is crucial and can hardly be evaluated by pre-therapeutic imaging. Furthermore, the size (e.g. the volume) of the lesion must be within the limits of radiosurgery which are also correlated with patients' condition and lesion topography. Clinicians are used to measure the diameter of the lesion and historically consider a diameter of 3 cm as the upper size limitation for a radiosurgical procedure. However, radiosurgeons prefer to take into account the volume of the lesion, which is a more suitable risk predictor in photon radiosurgery [1]. Furthermore, tumor volume may serve as a quantitative outcome parameter. No general size limitation can be suggested. It depends on the specific circumstances in each individual case such as location and configuration of the lesion, pre-treatment procedure (surgery, radiation therapy), and multimodality management like additional endovascular treatments or chemotherapy.

Standardized treatment cycle

A standardized treatment cycle is the basis for a successful radiosurgical procedure. There are four basic components of the gamma knife surgery procedure: 1. frame application, 2. stereotactic imaging, 3. treatment planning, 4. radiation delivery.

Duration of the procedure varies with type and size of lesion and decay of the ^{60}Co radiation sources. The larger and more complex the target, the longer the procedure time.

The initial part of the procedure is the application of the stereotactic frame. Immobilization of the head and its contained target by a stereotactic frame is crucial for the accuracy of both imaging and treatment planning and positioning during treatment. The frame provides a common reference base for imaging with fiducial markers and fixation to the treatment device. During the infiltration of local anaesthetics, blood pressure and pulse are regularly monitored by cuff readings. In anxious patients a mild sedation might be indicated. The position of the frame is crucial. It is important to position the frame on patient's head in a way that the targeted lesion is moved toward the frame center. The screws must be fixed tight to the skull to avoid any movement of the frame but penetration of the tabula externa has to be avoided. After attachment of the frame, the patient is examined by stereotactic imaging. All patients receive an MRI scan as basic imaging procedure and an additional CT scan or digital angiography if indicated. In Munich a 1.0 Tesla MRI scanner (Expert, Siemens Medical solutions, Erlangen, Germany) is used with a long and narrow gantry to establish a homogeneous magnetic field [8, 7]. Over ten years, this assured a stable overall accuracy of the Munich Radiosurgical System (MRS) of less than 0.5 mm [6]. It is important that the responsible radiosurgeon supervises the whole imaging procedure. Standard imaging sequences include 3-D MPR, 3-D CISS and T2-weighted imaging. No regular CT scanning is performed. CT is supplementary to MRI only for selected lesions in very critical areas. Images are sent to the Gamma-Plan workstation via a local network. The first step of dose planning is to analyse the stereotactic images with respect to imaging quality. The second step is to identify the number of targets and the individual risk organs. For this purpose, the specific features of the GammaPlan software (e.g. image correlation, image fusion, dose-volume histograms) have proven to be very useful. Risk organs are the optical apparatus, the brain stem, cranial nerves, pituitary gland, and the microvasculature in specific brain regions (for example the mesial temporal lobe).

The appropriate dose level is dependent on the tolerance doses of specific cranial structures: for example the facial nerve in tumors of the cerebello-pontine angle or the oculomotor nerves in skull base meningiomas. Another example are treatment strategies in pituitary adenomas. In secretory pituitary adenomas the cure of endocrinopathy is the major goal of therapy. Therefore, these tumors require higher doses than non-secretory adenomas. The tolerance doses for the specific neural structures are given in Table 1.

Risk organs and targets both are completely outlined in the image stack containing them in order to measure the corresponding volumes. Outlining is mandatory for all types of targets except some arteriovenous malformations and cases with multiple small spherical metastases. For dose planning, the multiple-isocenter principle is used. Regarding the number of isocenters per lesion a certain standard has been developed: benign tumors are treated by approximately four isocentre positions per cm^3 of tumor volume and malignant lesions by one, respectively. With this standard the dose to the target is appropriately concentrated, the conformity meets the specific requirements, and the procedure time can be kept within reasonable limits. In general, the tumour border corresponds to the 50–65% isodose. In certain risky conditions, an asymmetrical dose gradient is generated. For example, in vestibular schwannoma the steepest dose decay is at the anterior tumor margin in order to spare the facial nerve. It has to be taken into account – for physical reasons – that this can be achieved only at the expense of a less steep dose gradient on the opposite side of the tumor.

Table 1. *Shows the dose limits for critical neural structures used in Munich during the last 10 years*

Optical nerve, chiasm	≤6 Gy
Oculomotor nerves	≤18 Gy
Trigeminal nerve	≤15 Gy
Facial nerve	≤13 Gy
Pituitary gland	≤15 Gy
Pons (surface dose)	≤15 Gy
Medulla oblongata	≤8 Gy
Mesial temporal lobe (5 cm^3)	≤10 Gy

This feature is similar to the inverse dose planning principle. The next part of dose planning is to prescribe the appropriate dose level. The dose level is determined by the type of lesion, its size and its location. In general, there is a dose-effect-relationship for radiation therapy. Moreover, there is a considerable biological heterogeneity in malignant and also in benign tumors. Because of these two aspects we aim to give the highest reasonable treatment dose in every individual case. This means that in malignant tumors (brain metastases), a high dose level of $D_{min} = 18–22$ Gy is applied while in benign tumors a considerably lower dose (12–18 Gy) is given. In this respect the so-called 10-Gy volume (volume of the non-targeted tissue which receives a minimum dose of 10-Gy), according to a more global definition than originally proposed by Voges *et al.* [12], is of concern as a parameter for the applied dose to the surrounding healthy brain tissue. Ob-

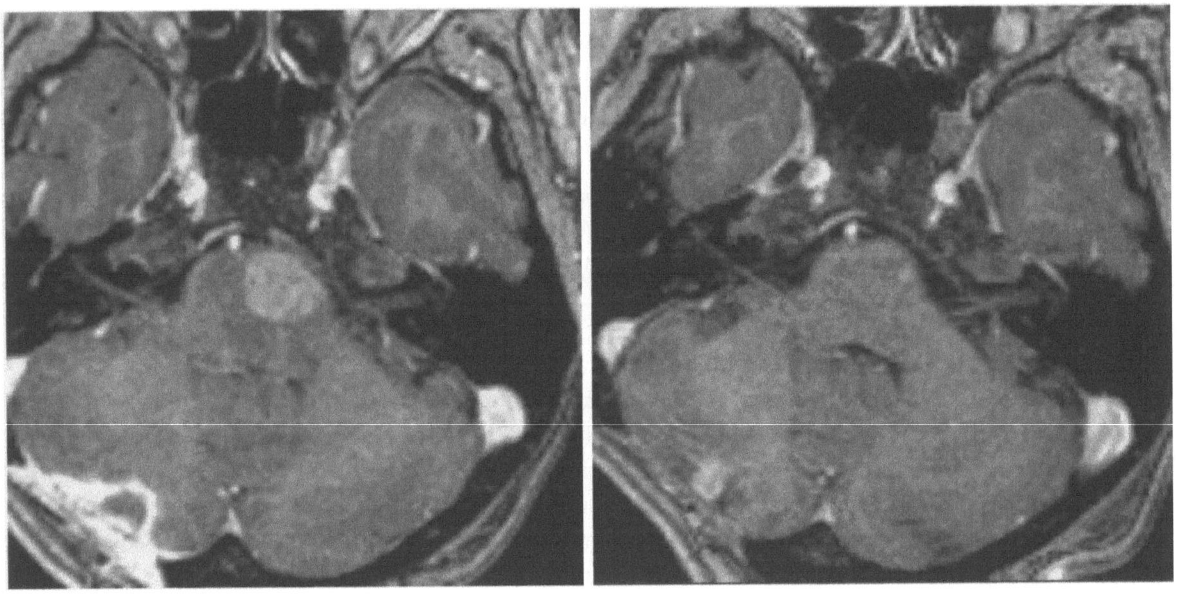

Fig. 2. This patient was treated microsurgically for a right cerebellar metastasis (left side). Four weeks after surgery a local recurrence was suspected and a new brain stem metastasis had developed. The suspected local recurrence was treated by a boost dose of 18 Gy and the brain stem with 20 Gy to the margin of the lesion. Five weeks after gamma knife radiosurgery (right side) both the recurrent lesion and the brain stem metastasis have successfully been treated

viously, the 10-Gy volume is larger in malignant than in benign targets because of a higher conformity index in benign lesions as outlined above. For example, in our vestibular schwannoma series ($n = 318$) the 10-Gy volume was rather small (median: 2.60 cm^3; range: 0.11 cm^3 to 21.4 cm^3) and was significantly correlated with the volume of the schwannomas (median: 1.50 cm^3; range: 0.03 cm^3 to 13.0 cm^3) ($p < 0.0001$, $r = 0.94$). In contrast, in malignant tumors, for example in cases of singular metastases ($n = 154$), the 10-Gy volume is much larger (median: 4.05 cm^3; range: 0.01 cm^3 to 40.6 cm^3). It is also significantly correlated with the volume of the metastases (median: 14.4 cm^3; range: 1.40 cm^3 to 118.10 cm^3) ($p < 0.0002$, $r = 0.93$). Regarding these measured values, one can estimate that the index between the volume of the lesion and the 10-Gy volume in cases of singular metastases ($14.4/4.05 = 3.56$) is double the corresponding index in vestibular schwannoma radiosurgery ($2.6/1.5 = 1.73$).

Integrated therapeutical concept

Gamma knife radiosurgery is ideally integrated in a multidisciplinary team. Such a team should consist of neurosurgeons with subspecialization in radiosurgery, neurosurgeons with subspecialization in skull base surgery and vascular neurosurgery, neuroradiologists/neurosurgeons with subspecialization in endovascular techniques, oncologists and radio-oncologists. The potential of gamma knife radiosurgery will only be maximized in a setting of close relation to a hospital managing the full range of neurosurgical indications. For example, skull base meningiomas are ideally treated by an interdisciplinary team consisting of neursurgeons subspecialized in skull base surgery and radiosurgeons. The surgeon has the possibility to reduce the main tumor mass until close to critical structures in order not to induce any neurological deficit. The part of tumor in proximity to critical structures like nerves and vessels will safely be treated by an experienced radiosurgeon. Another example would be a patient of good clinical grade with a stable systemic tumor status harboring brain metastases. Figure 2 is showing a case where a large cerebellar metastasis was treated microsurgically and an additional brainstem metastasis that occurred only shortly after surgery was treated by gamma knife radiosurgery.

Another example of an interdisciplinary treatment concept is the treatment of arteriovenous malformations (AVM). AVMs are frequently treated by a combination of endovascular embolization and micro-

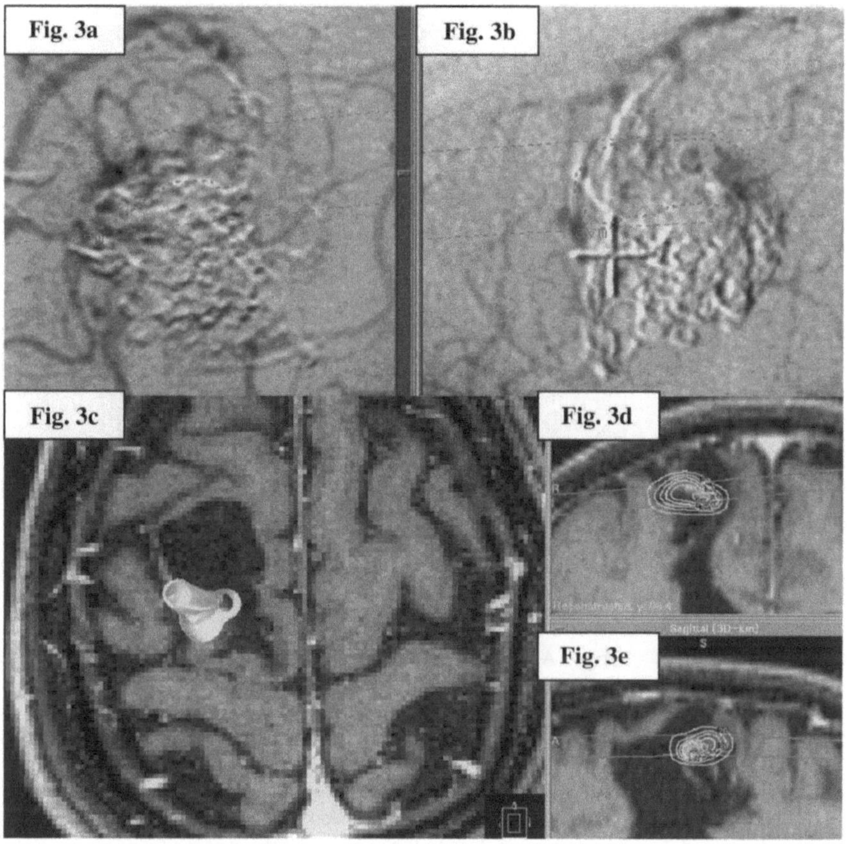

Fig. 3. A right sided precentral AVM treated by endovascular embolization and gamma knife radiosurgery of the vascular remnants of the upper dorsal aspects of the lesion. Figure 3a and b are displaying two sequences of the DSA with overlay of the outline of radiosurgery treatment volume. Figure 3c is showing the 3-D reconstruction of the treatment volume and figures 3d and e are depicting the coronal and sagittal view of the planned isodoses and the overlay of DSA localization

surgery. Small AVMs can be treated by radiosurgery alone or in combination with endovascular and/or microsurgery. Embolization can be beneficial for radiosurgery if it leads to a definite volume reduction, thereby allowing a smaller volume to be targeted for radiosurgery. The accuracy of radiosurgical treatment of AVMs is dependent on the accuracy of target delineation by radiological studies performed with the stereotactic frame in place. For treatment planning of vascular malformations a stereotactic three dimensional subtraction angiography (DSA) today is a diagnostic standard and should be performed immediately before radiosurgery. In order to achieve highest possible localization accuracy and to fully understand the three-dimensional topographic and tomographic anatomy of the malformation as well as the relationship between the targeted AVM and the non-targeted anatomical structures of the AVM, the DSA should be fused and overlaid on the pretreatment MRI (Fig. 3). Treatment planning comprises target outlines marked on the angiogram to be projeceted on the MRIs and vice versa. Adding another dimension to such planning ensures better coverage of the target. A three-dimensional representation of the target can then be used to assess the plan. The importance of using both angiography and MRI data is underscored.

Specific treatment characteristics

Conformity/concentration

Radiosurgery depends fundamentally on precisely tailored radiation delivery. Recent improvements of radiosurgical imaging, computer hardware and software, and stereotactic radiation delivery systems have made it possible to tailor the delivery of radiation to an unprecedented degree [2, 3, 4]. By using these techno-

Table 2. *Gives the prescription dose levels and the isodoses used by the authors for various lesions*

	D_{MD} [Gy]	D_{min} [Gy]	D_{max} [Gy]	ISODOSE [%]
Trigeminalneuralgia	85	75	85	100
AV-malformation	23	18	25	50
Acoustic neurinoma	12.5	11.5	13.5	50
Meningioma	16	13	17	50
Cerebral metastases	19	17	22	>50

MD Mean dose, *Dmin* minimum target dose, *Dmax* maximum target dose.

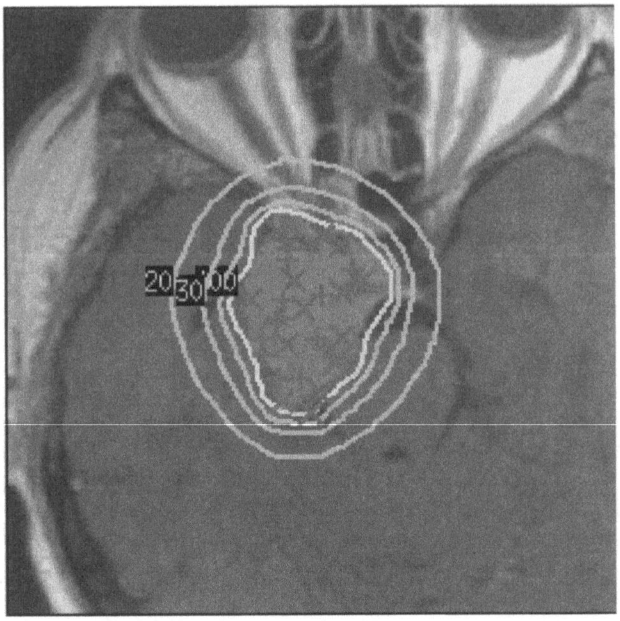

Fig. 4. A twenty-five isocenter complex planning for a cavernous sinus meningioma. Through methodological application of the techniques and principles described above, highly conformal treatment plans can be achieved for even the most complex lesions. The plan includes 25 isocenters of various shapes and sizes. Note the conformality of the prescription isodose line to the contour of the tumor. A dose of 16 Gy was prescribed to the 50% isodose shell. The maximum dose to the optic apparatus was <7 Gy

logical advances, radiosurgeons are improving efficacy and diminishing complications. A steep dose gradient at the boundary of the target is critical because a single high dose of radiation is delivered with the intention of killing all neoplastic tissue included in the target volume. The more its marginal dose matches the contours of the target and, simultaneously, the steeper the dose gradient, the higher the effective dose to the target. Using this principle, the exposure of non-targeted tissue is minimised. The degree to which a planned volume of radiation conforms to the radiographically targeted volume depends on the physical aspects of the radiation used and the delivery device. The gamma knife does this by using multiple exposures dispersed throughout a target volume and up to 201 beams per exposure. The beams are precisely focused on a selected target resulting in a very high relative target dose and a steep dose gradient outside the target (dose concentration). This method of summing dose contributions from many beams of radiation at one target is the basis of radiosurgery.

Dose gradient/tolerance

In the case of an adjacent highly radiosensitive, critical neural structure the dose gradient has to be optimized. The optic apparatus and the brain stem are of highest concern, as these are the most sensitive structures of the brain. Selection of an appropriate dose for a given lesion is obviously critical to safe and effective radiosurgical treatment (Table 2). Lowering doses may be indicated in case of a pre-existing neurological deficit and in patients who have undergone prior radiation treatment.

The critical task is generally to gain an overview of the lesion configuration and its location relative to highly radiosensitive neurological tissue (Fig. 4). Expertise and persistence during the iterative process of designing complex plans is essential for successful multiple-isocenter treatment planning.

Patient follow-up

It is important to standardize the dosimetric parameters so that a consistent pattern of treatment can be followed and coherent statements can be formulated regarding the clinical response to a given treatment regime. In this regard a regular clinical and imaging follow-up must be regarded as extremely important. The specific clinical and imaging features after radiosurgery should be evaluated and interpreted by the radiosurgeon who performed the procedure, otherwise misinterpretation of these features can easily occur. For example, frequently a clinical increase of neurological symptoms may be seen in the early phase after radiosurgery. This is often correlated with an increase of perifocal edema which in most cases can be treated by a short course of steroids. Ideally all follow-up imaging is done at the same institution were the ra-

Table 3. *Sequential tumor volumetry of a reference vestibular schwannoma after gamma knife surgery. The values are descriptive statistics of 10 measurements at every examination date*

Examination date (months after GKS)	Median (cm^3)	Mean (cm^3)	Mean (% of T_0)	SD	Min.	Max.	Percentage SD
0.0	1.30	1.28	100%	0.06	1.20	1.40	4.9%
3.4	1.60*	1.58*	123%	0.08	1.50	1.70	5.0%
9.4	2.30*	2.30*	180%*	0.16	2.00	2.50	7.1%
21.4	1.10	1.14	89%	0.07	1.10	1.30	6.3%
34.2	0.42	0.42	33%	0.03	0.36	0.46	7.4%
47.3	0.29	0.27	21%	0.05	0.19	0.33	17.1%
69.3	0.16	0.16	12%	0.02	0.12	0.19	13.6%

SD Standard deviation, T_0 Date of GKS, * Indicates VS swelling.

diosurgical procedure is performed. In the German Gamma Knife Center Munich the aim is to perform follow-up imaging at the same scanner where radiosurgical MRI planning was done. All images are then sent to the planning computer workstation where a volumetric calculation of the lesion is performed. Tumor volumetry is a standard for description of the quantitative treatment results. A quantitative follow-up volumetry is the most exact imaging based outcome parameter and has its particular value in the definition of treatment results of benign lesions. Regular follow-up volumetry allows the definition of dynamic imaging changes (Table 3).

This allows an exact monitoring of the induced biological and imaging related effects. Particularly the specific tissue characteristics deserve a thorough evaluation because only an experienced radiosurgeon can interpret the specific imaging changes in a meaningful way. Enlargement represents either true neoplastic tumor growth or tumor death with an expansion of the tumor margins as the central portion of the tumor is inactivated. In the latter case, subsequent imaging studies are important to confirm tumor volume regression (Fig. 5).

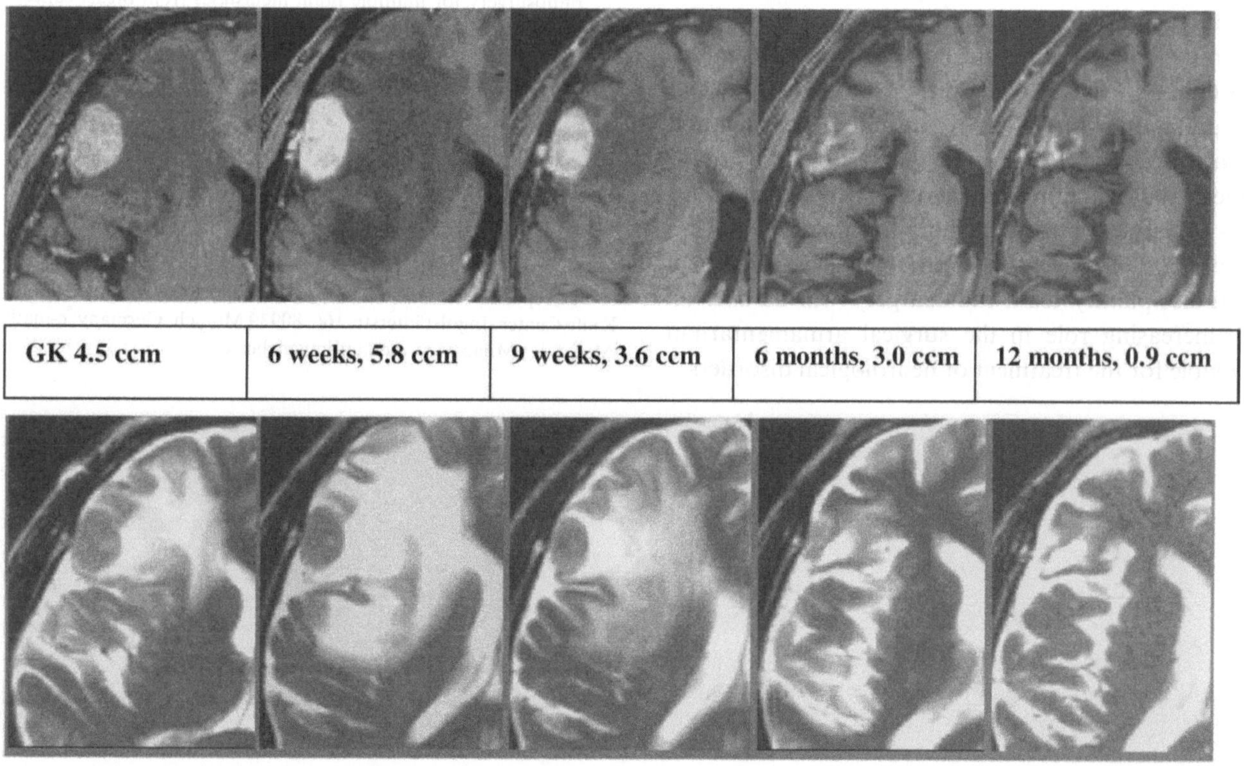

Fig. 5. Depicts the treatment effects after gamma knife radiosurgery in a patient harboring a singular right frontal metastasis of a malignant melanoma. In the upper row the T_1-weighted contrast enhanced imaging and in the lower row the corresponding T_2-weighted imaging are displayed. At the time of treatment the tumor had a volume of 4.5 ccm. After six weeks there was an enlargement of the lesion (5.8 ccm) and the perifocal edema. Nine weeks after radiosurgery there was a continuous reduction of the tumor volume and associated edema. Six months and one year after treatment only residual tumor aspects are seen

Scientific data analysis

Gamma knife radiosurgery has been demonstrated to play a significant therapeutic role in the management of new or recurrent intracranial lesions. Furthermore it has a growing impact on residual tumors after microsurgical treatment and functional indications. By standardizing treatment protocols and reporting requirements for scientific publications of clinical results, continued progress can be made to define optimal techniques and the role of radiosurgical management in these lesions [9, 10]. Therefore it is of utmost importance to perform a regular data evaluation, ideally in form of a prospective protocol. Particularly the specific complications after radiosurgery must be meticulously monitored and documented to gain information not only on induced treatment effects but also on clinical limitations in each individual case. In the authors' institution all patient treatment and follow-up data are stored on an electronic computerized data base. These data can rapidly be checked and compared to similar cases. Moreover a quick overview of the statistics like local tumor control rate or survival times can easily be calculated by conveying the electronically stored data directly to a statistics program. This rapid insight into the own data collection enables a 'state of the art' data evaluation and interpretation without time consuming investigation of patient charts. Emphazing long-term follow-up in clinical trials will ultimately allow to define the relative roles of surgical resection, radiation therapy, and radiosurgery. However, the authors believe that in a multi-disciplinary team radiosurgery will assume an ever-increasing role in the surgical armamentarium available for the treatment of neurological disorders.

References

1. Arndt J. Focussed Gamma Radiation. The gamma knife (1993) In: Phillips MH (ed) Physical aspects of stereotactic radiosurgery. Plenum Press, New York, pp 87–128
2. Flickinger JC (1989) An integrated logistic formula for prediction of complications from radiosurgery. Int J Radiat Oncol Biol Phys 17: 879–885
3. Flickinger JC, Lunsford LD, Wu A *et al* (1990) Treatment planning for gamma knife radiosurgery with multiple isocenters. Int J Oncol Biol Phys 18: 1495–1501
4. Foote, KD, Friedman WA, Meeks SL *et al* (1999) Radiosurgical software and dose planning. Linac and gamma knife radiosurgery. In: Germano IM (ed) AANS, USA, p 31–55
5. Leksell L (1951) The stereotactic method of and radiosurgery of the brain. Acta Chir Scand 102: 316–319
6. Mack A, Czempiel H, Kreiner HJ *et al* (2002) Quality assurance in stereotactic space. A system test for verifying the accuracy of aim in radiosurgery. Med Phys 29: 561–568
7. Mack A, Mack G, Weltz D (2003) Quality assurance in stereotactic space. Determination of the accuracy of aim and dose in single dose radiosurgery. Strahlenther Onkol 179: 760–766
8. Mack A, Wolff R, Weltz D (2002) Experimentally determined three-dimensional dose distributions in small complex targets. J Neurosurg 97: 551–555
9. Muacevic A, Kreth FW, Horstmann GA *et al* (1999) Surgery and radiotherapy compared with gamma knife radiosurgery in the treatment of solitary cerebral metastases of small diameter. J Neurosurg 91: 35–43
10. Muacevic A, Kreth FW, Tonn JC, Wowra B (2004) Stereotactic radiosurgery for multiple brain metastases from breast cancer: feasibility and outcome of a local treatment concept. Cancer 15: 1705–1711
11. Stiebler VW, Bourland JD, Thome WL, Mehta MM (2003) Gentlemen (and Ladies), choose your weapons: Gamma Knife vs. linear accelerator radiosurgery. Techn Cancer Res Treat 2: 79–85
12. Voges J, Treuer H, Sturm V *et al* (1996) Risk analysis of linear accelerator radiosurgery. Int J Radiat Oncol Biol Phys 36: 1055–1063

Correspondence: Alexander Muacevic, M.D., German Gamma Knife Center, Ingolstädterstr. 166, 80939 Munich, Germany. e-mail: Alexander.Muacevic@med.uni-muenchen.de

Acta Neurochir (2004) [Suppl] 91: 33–50

Gamma knife surgery for epilepsy related to hypothalamic hamartomas

J. Régis[1], M. Hayashi[1], L. P. Eupierre[1], N. Villeneuve[2], F. Bartolomei[2], T. Brue[2], and P. Chauvel[2]

[1] Stereotactic and Functional Neurosurgery Department, Timone Hospital, Marseilles, France
[2] Endocrinology Department, Timone Hospital, Marseilles, France

Summary

Objective. Drug resistant epilepsy associated with hypothalamic hamartoma (HH) can be cured by microsurgical resection of the lesion. Morbidity and mortality risks of microsurgery in this area are significant. Gamma Knife Surgery's (GKS) reduced invasivity seems to be well adapted. In view of the severity of the disease and risks of surgical resection it is crucial to evaluate GKS for this indication. A first retrospective study has shown a very good safety and efficacy level but for a more reliable evaluation a prospective study would be required.

Methods. Between Oct 1999 and July 2002, 30 patients with HH and associated severe epilepsy were included. Seizure semiology (video EEG) and frequency, behavioural disturbances, neuropsychological performance, endocrinological status, sleep electroclinical abnormalities, MR imaging, and visual function were systematically evaluated before and after GKS (6, 12, 18, 24, 36 months). Twenty patients had experienced precocious puberty at a median age of 3,7 (0–9). Range of maximum diameter was from 7,5 to 23 mm with only 3 larger than 18 mm. The median marginal dose was 17 gy (14–20).

Results. Sufficient follow up for final evaluation is not yet available. Only 6 patients have a follow-up of more than 12 months and 19 more than 6 months. However a lot of very dramatic changes did occur during that period in this group. Among the 19 patients with more than 6 months of follow-up, a lot had already experienced an increase of gelastic seizures around 3 months (3), an improvement in their seizure rate (18), behaviour (9), sleep (3), and EEG background activity (3), a cessation of partial complex seizures (7). No complications have occurred till now except one patient experiencing at 5 months a hyperthermia without infection and concomitant increase of gelastic seizures both ceasing suddenly and spontaneously after 15 days.

Conclusion. Our first results indicate that GKS is as effective as microsurgical resection and very much safer. GKS also allows to avoid the vascular risk related to radiofrequency lesioning or stimulation. The disadvantage of radiosurgery is its delayed action. Longer follow-up is mandatory for a serious evaluation of the role of GKS. Results are faster and more complete in patients with smaller lesions inside the 3rd ventricle (grade II). The early effect on subclinical discharges turns out to play a major role in the dramatic improvement of sleep quality, behaviour, developmental acceleration at school.

Keywords: Behaviour disorder; epilepsy surgery; gamma knife radiosurgery; gelastic seizures; hypothalamic hamartomas; precocious puberty.

Introduction

What is radiosurgery?

Radiosurgery is a neurosurgical procedure where converging narrow ionizing beams are stereotactically focussed in order to induce a desired biological effect in a predetermined target, with minimal radiation to the surrounding tissues and without opening the skull. A Swedish neurosurgeon, Lars Leksell, in 1951, was the first to introduce this concept of radiosurgery. His goal was to perform stereotactic procedures without opening the skull in order to avoid bleeding and infection risks.

General results of radiosurgery

Safety/efficacy of radiosurgery has well been demonstrated in numerous indications such as arteriovenous malformations [39, 74], vestibular schwannomas [30, 48, 58], metastasis [23, 25, 42, 71], pituitary adenomas [16, 36, 57], meningiomas [31, 69]. Obviously, as soon as resection of a small lesion deeply seated is considered a risk for surgical complications and/or functional worsening, gamma knife surgery must be discussed. For these indications GKS compares favorably with microsurgical removal in terms of safety/efficacy but also cost-effectiveness. Enormous experience has been gained worldwide using GKS in various indications rendering the side effects of radiosurgery rare, generally transient and quite easily predictable [22].

Rationale for the use of radiosurgery in epilepsy surgery

These advantages of GKS, namely high safety and efficacy, comfort, very short hospital stay (2 nights) the immediate capability of the patient to go back to work at the former activity level are very appealing for functional neurosurgery in general, and epilepsy surgery in particular.

In addition, the use of GKS in various pathological conditions has revealed a likely specific antiepileptic effect when applied to patients with severe epilepsy as an associated condition (for review see [60]). Finally, in a homogeneous group of patients with mesial temporal lobe epilepsies (MTLE) we have demonstrated the short-middle term safety and efficiency of GK surgery in this indication [62, 63]. The responsibility of HH in the genesis of seizures was first suggested by the successful resection of HH itself in some patients [49, 56] but direct demonstration of the role of HH was provided by the data obtained during stereo-EEG recordings. These studies demonstrated initial ictal discharges in the HH during gelastic or dacrystic seizures [29]. However, in this critical area, microsurgical resection of HH entails a very high risk of complications, including oculomotor palsy, hemiparesis, and visual field deficit [17]. Arita *et al.* in 1999 reported a first case of successful treatment by gamma knife surgery with no side effect [4].

Retrospective analysis

Based on this rationale, and considering the key role of HH in the genesis and treatment of associated epilepsy, we have considered the potential role of GKS for this very specific epileptic condition. We have experience with radiosurgery in the area of the hypothalamus for different kinds of pathologies which allows us to predict the risks and to evaluate the technical requirements for safety. However, in this essentially pediatric population we have considered it mandatory to first analyse the rare cases already treated worldwide and then to treat the new patients in the scope of a multicenter prospectively controlled trial. As a consequence we have recently reported on the results of a retrospective multicenter study which is in fact the first series evaluating the efficacy and morbidity of GK radiosurgery in this indication [59]. The 8 patients included had severe drug resistant epilepsy as main expression and 3 patients had precocious puberty. All were drug resistant and presented generalized seizures and partial complex seizures suggesting the involvement of temporal and/or frontal cortex in addition to simple gelastic and/or dacrystic seizures. Two patients had a previous history of unsuccessful partial microsurgical resection. Two patients were treated twice (second GKS at 19 and 49 months after the first one) due to insufficient efficacy of the first procedure. Median follow-up was 28 months after GKS (range 12–71; mean 35). All patients were improved. Four patients were seizure free (one with residual auras), one had rare nocturnal seizures , one had some rare partial seizures and no more generalized attacks, and two were improved only with a reduction in seizure frequency but still had some rare generalized seizures. However, minor gelastic, complex partial and atypical absence of seizures persisted in 4 patients, although at significantly reduced rates, but there has been a dramatic improvement in behaviour and cognition. Median latency in seizure cessation was 9 months (mean 14,25; range 3 to 36 months). No side effect was reported except for one patient who presented a non-disabling poïkilothermia. The excellent safety rate for an efficacy similar to microsurgical resection demonstrated in this series has led us to organize a prospective study.

Materials and methods

The presurgical work-up included a neurological, neurosurgical and ophthalmological assessment. All patients underwent a video EEG recording of seizures, high resolution MR imaging including coronal T2 weighted images and FLAIR sequences. Systematically a detailed clinical and biological endocrine evaluation was performed before radiosurgery. Neuropsychological testing and psychiatric evaluation were adapted to age, behaviour and eventual mental retardation. The preoperative cognitive deficits, behavioural disturbances and investigated relationship of seizure severity and anatomical type to cognitive abilities were characterized [24, 83]. Ictal and interictal SPECT were available for some patients but not mandatory. The goal of the preoperative work-up was to adequately select the candidates for inclusion and to evaluate the baseline neurological and endocrinological functions.

All radiosurgical procedures were carried out using the Leksell 201-source Cobalt 60 gamma knife (Elekta Instrument, Stockholm) [37, 38]. Patients were admitted to hospital the night before the operation. Radiosurgery was performed under local anesthesia or under general anesthesia for younger children. Children returned home at their preoperative level of function within 1 day after treatment. Adults were not anesthetized and returned to their preoperative level of function immediately. On the morning of the treatment an imaging-compatible stereotactic coordinate frame (Elekta Instrument) was applied to the patient's head. We then performed a high resolution stereotactic MR and Ct scan.

Radiosurgical technique

Images were sent directly through the local network on dedicated workstations allowing concomitant navigation in stereotactic images and calculation of three dimensional planning of the radiosurgery (GammaPlan software, Elekta Instrument, Stockholm, Sweden). On the MR the boundaries of HH were cautiously identified relying

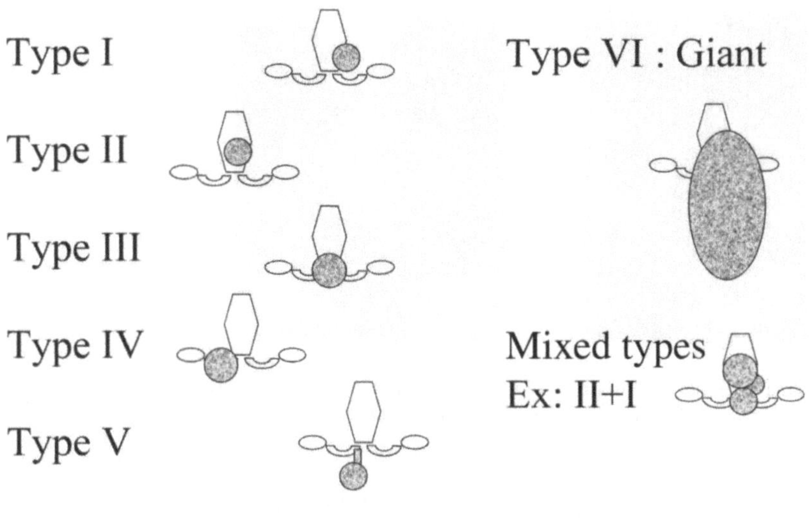

Type	I	II & III	IV	V	VI
Main site	Hypothalamus	Third ventricle (II) or floor (III)	Under floor sessile	Under floor pediculate	Giant including several sites
Epilepsy	yes	yes	yes	no (very rare)	yes
Precocious puberty	rare	possible	possible	frequent	frequent
Cognitive impairement	+/−	+/−	+++	0	++++
Behavioural abnormalities	+/−inhibition	+/−aggressivity hyperkinetic	+++inhibition	0	++++aggressivity hyperkinetic
Surgery	gamma knife	1 gamma knife 2 endoscopic 3 transcallosal 4 susoptic	if big pterional if small GK	medical trt if epilepsy GK or pterional	combination pterional + transcallosal GK on remnant

Fig. 1. Topological Classification of Hypothalamic Hamartomas: Classification of hypothalamic hamartomas into these 6 categories based on MR findings resulted in a clear correlation between symptoms and the subsequent clinical course (IV versus the others) and is pertinent for clinical management. We speculate that sessile hypothalamic hamartomas have always more or less an «extension» in the hypothalamus close to the mammilary body. Thus when a lesion is classified as a type II, that means that the lesion appears on the MR like mainly located in the third ventricle but is likely to have a «root» in the hypothalamus. The same assumption is made for type III. In the table associated with the figure the more frequent clinical pattern reported for each anatomical type is noted and our actual therapeutic management strategy indicated

on axial and coronal T2 high resolution images. At the same stage boundaries and relationship with HH of the surrounding critical structures including mamillary bodies, fornices (on axial T2), tuber cinereum, pituitary stalk, optic tract, chiasm, and nerve were analysed. Tomographic imaging scans are complementary to MRI imaging and allow verification of a lack of distortion in the latter. Consistently we elaborated multi isocentric complex dose planning of high conformity and selectivity. However, some limited part of the HH were deliberately left uncovered as soon as a more complete coverage was supposed to increase functional risk. The 50% isodose line was used to match the lesion margin in most patients. We used low peripheral doses to take into account the close relationship with optic pathways and hypothalamus (Fig. 2). The median dose at the marginal isodose was 17 Gy (range: 14 to 20 Gy; mean 16,73). The median value of the maximal diameter of HH was 13,5 mm (range 8–23; mean 13,7). The median volume of the marginal isodose was 646,7 mm^3 (range 134–2674,8; mean 889,4). The mean number of isocenters used for each procedure was 20 isocenters/treatment (range 4–36; median 10,5). Beam blocking strategy was frequently used in this indication in order to improve the steep fall-off of dose gradient at the marginal parts of the lesion in close relation to the optic pathways. Systematically parts of the HH too close to the optic pathways were uncovered (figure 1). A threshold of 10 Gy to the optic tract and 8 Gy to the chiasm and nerve was respected in each case. The median maximum dose delivered to the optic tract was 6,4 Gy (mean 7,6; range 3–12,2), to the optic chiasm was 3,8 Gy (mean 4,9 Gy; range 1–5, 8,3 Gy), to the optic nerve was 2,8 (mean 4,65; range 0,8–8,5). The median maximum dose to the mammillary bodies was 19,66 Gy (mean 18,75; range 5,3–32,2 Gy). Patients were evaluated with respect to seizures, cognition, behaviour, and endocrine status 6, 12, 18 and 24 months after radiosurgery.

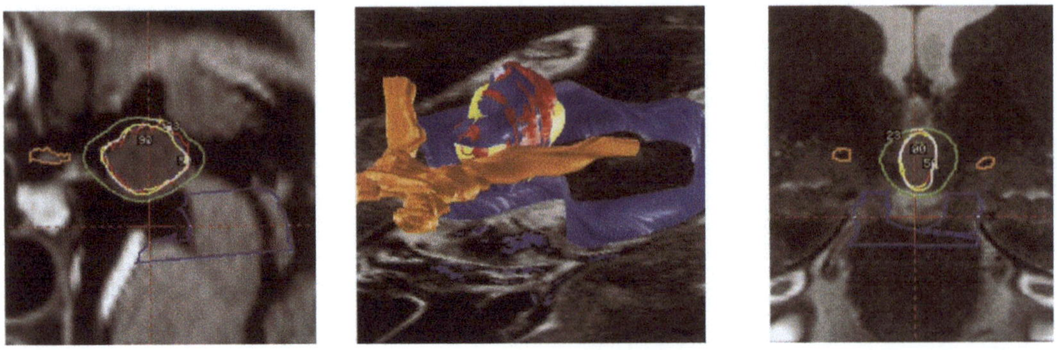

Fig. 2. Dosemetry of a type II hypothalamic hamartoma. The marginal isodose (17 Gy) is displayed in yellow. The green line corresponds to the 23% isodose line (7,82 Gy) and is sparing the optic pathways illustrating the very good fall off of the dose gradient

Results

Population

The final study population for the prospective trial was composed of 30 patients. Two patients already included have not yet been treated. Median age was 15,9 years (range: 3–40; mean 17,9) at the time of GKS. Three of these patients had previously been operated microsurgically in other centers and were then referred to us due to insufficient results on seizures. One of these patients experienced severe postoperative complications including hemiplegia, appetite stimulation with severe obesity, blindness of one eye and important visual loss on the other. This patient presented initially with a large type III HH (see Fig. 1). Resection performed microsurgically was minimal and clinically very deleterious. The other two patients were operated subtotally with no surgical complication and only a very small remnant corresponding to the small part directly in the hypothalamus. No parenchymal damage was visible in the surrounding tissue on the stereotactic MRI (including flair sequence). In spite of the very extensive removal via susoptic approach one patient still had a lot of seizures even if this one of the two patients undoubtedly was improved by resection (and was even seizure free postoperatively for several months). Owing to the quality of resection and since no injury to the surrounding critical structures had occurred, radiosurgery had not been complexified by the previous resection. In all these cases diagnosis of HH was based on an MR examination including T1 before and after gadolinium injection and T2 weighted sequences. All patients except one had sessile HH corresponding to the Valdueza type IIA and IIB [81]. According to Valdueza [81], type II corresponds to medium/large sessile HH broadly attached to the tuber cinereum or mamillary body [81], the absence (IIA) or presence (IIB) of mass effect on the hypothalamus distinguishing the two subgroups (IIA and IIB). In this study, we chose to classify these lesions according to an original classification, more adapted, in the authors opinion, to the anatomy of this region as well as the clinical patterns of presentation and therapeutic management (see Fig. 1). Eleven were essentially located in the hypothalamus either with no extension (class I = 4) or only just a shallowing mesially in the 3rd ventricle (I + II = 5) or an extension below the floor of the ventricle (III = 2). Twelve were essentially in the 3rd ventricle with only a small extension into the hypothalamus (Class II + I = 9) or no lesion clearly visible in the hypothalamus (class II = 3). Three were essentially below the floor of the 3rd ventricle either with no main extension in the hypothalamus (class III = 2) or with a clear involvement of the hypothalamus (class III + I = 1). Only 1 was pediculated (class IV) with no lesion visible in the hypothalamus. No lesion was giant (class V). The very big lesions were excluded according to the inclusion criterion of the protocol. The median of the maximum diameter was 11,7 (mean 16,1; range 7,2–25). In two patients the important size of the lesion led us to propose as first intention a partial treatment confined to the upper part of the lesion. For both the recommended microsurgical resection had been refused by the family. In all the patients the lesion was in very close relation to the mammillary body.

Semiology

Preoperatively, all patients had a history of variable combinations of gelastic, complex partial and generalized seizures resistant to two or more antiepileptic drugs. Median age at seizure onset for gelastic seizures was 5,23 months (range 0–228; mean 29). Generalized seizures were reported in 18 patients (60%) and the median age of onset for this type of seizures was 95,2 months (mean 110,9 months; range 19,6–312,3). All presented partial complex seizures suggesting the involvement of temporal and or frontal cortex in addition to simple gelastic and or dacrystic seizures. The median of onset of the partial complex seizures was 67,3 months (mean 0–228,28 months; range 63,7). In 8 patients an epileptic status had been reported (median age 148,5 months). None of the patients were subjected to depth electrode recording. Median frequency of seizure prior to GK was 41,83 episodes/month (range 3–1560; mean 257,53). In only 4 of these 30 patients (13,3%) the semiology of the seizures was starting by gelastic phenomenon (or equivalent) at the time of radiosurgery.

Four patients had overweight. The growth hormone peak, free thyroxine, cortisol and prolactin concentrations, and the concomitant plasma and urinary osmolalities were normal in all cases evaluated (except two of the patients who had previously been operated microsurgically and one patient with no previous surgery but a slightly low T3–T4 from hypothalamic origin).

Effect on behaviour and cognitive functions

Mental retardation was present in 30% of the patients. IQ was of a low average in an additional 26% and in the normal range in 44%. Long term retrieval was poor in 29%. Processing speed was low in 60%. A relative strength of visual processing as compared to verbal was observed in 33% of the patients.

In this group of patients we observed a high rate of psychiatric co-morbidity. Generally, selective sustained attention and control of impulsivity are poor. A significant increase in aggression behaviour was noticed in the majority of patients (60%). Most had an affective subtype of aggression [83]. Anxiety and mood disorder was observed in 43%, speech retardation/learning impairment in 50%, conduct disorder 54% clear attention-deficit and hyperactivity disorder in 54%, marked oppositional defiant disorder in 43%. Market inhibition was clear in 37%. A past history of hallucinations was reported by the referring physician in 13%.

On the basis of parental reports and our own subjective observations, the children exhibited marked improvements in behaviour, school performance, and quality of life. All these patients, except one (who was a failure for seizure control) have improved their behaviour. In 9 of these patients improvement was dramatic. Especially all the patients with paroxystic aggressivity improved substantially. Some of the patients more on the side of the inhibition had improved (70%) with increased alertness, elevated mood and greater speak production. Dramatic developmental acceleration was observed in 3 young patients.

Effect on sleep

Was frequently reported by the parents, mainly in the younger patients.

All patients with frequent interictal spikewaves on background EEG, except one had these abnormalities very much improved and normal EEG sleep pattern re-emerged in the months following radiosurgery.

Effects on seizures

For final evaluation sufficient follow-up is not yet available. Only 6 patients have a follow-up of more than 12 months and 19 more than 6 months. However, a lot of important changes occurred during that period in this group. Among the 19 patients with more than 6 months follow-up a lot had already experienced a transient increase of gelastic seizures around 3 months (3), an improvement in their seizure rate (18), and normalisation of the EEG background activity (3), a cessation of partial complex seizures (7) or even of the gelastic seizures (2). The patient partially treated was a complete failure and was operated microsurgically by an expert but unfortunately is not seizure free and experienced no cognitive or behavioural improvement. According to our experience with radiosurgery in this group of patients, first results can be evaluated in 2 years only.

Effects on precocious puberty

Twenty of the 30 patients had a past history of precocious puberty. All were safely and successfully treated by GnRH analog treatment. Only 2 of these 20 were treated early enough to judge the effect of radiosurgery concerning these symptoms. Median age of onset of precocious puberty was 5,6 years (range 0–9; mean 4,7). According to the protocol luteinizing hormone-releasing hormone analog (GnRH analog) treatment is supposed to be stopped 24 months after radiosurgery in order to evaluate the effect of GKS on precocious puberty. None of the two children has reached this point yet.

Safety (endocrinological, visual, neuropsychological)

No clinical or biological endocrine changes were observed. Especially no appetite stimulation or weight gain was reported, no thyroxyne blood level lowering, no hypernatremia.

No worsening of the cognitive abilities was observed. Especially no short term memory complaints were reported.

No new visual acuity or visual field deficits have been observed. No diplopia and above all no deterioration of the third nerve function. No neurological worsening was reported at any moment of the follow-up. No complications occurred till now except one patient experiencing at 5 months a hyperthermia without infection concomitant with an increase of gelastic seizures, both ceasing suddenly and spontaneously after 15 days. No patients presented reactional edema. None of the patients exhibited intracranial hypertension signs. MR scans performed at 6, 12, 18 and 24 months have demonstrated the absence of any changes even on the FLAIR sequences.

Discussion

Rationale for treatment by gamma knife surgery

Intrinsec Epileptogenicity of HH has been demonstrated even though the mechanisms of epilepsy associated with HH are still a matter of discussion. Hypothalamic hamartomas are heterotopic lesions composed of neurons, glia and myelinated fibers [49]. Resections of temporal or frontal lobe cortex [10] in patients investigated with intracranial electrodes and demonstrating tonic early involvement of these cortical areas have systematically failed to cure epilepsy. Moreover, pathological examination of resected cortex supposed to be epileptogenic did not reveal any abnormalities [10]. Responsibility of HH in the genesis of seizures was first suggested by successful resection of the HH itself in some patients (see above). Direct proof of the role of HH was provided by Munari relying on data obtained from stereo-EEG recordings [29, 43, 77]. In patients with gelastic [43] or dacrystic [29] seizures, a low-voltage fast recruiting discharge was first recorded in the HH before changes appeared in the other regions explored. This evidence was reinforced by ictal SPECT studies [20, 32, 33] and other studies using depth electrodes [5, 8]. Finally several Spectro-MR studies found the relative intensity of N-acetylaspartate to creating (NAA/Cr) and NAA/choline (Ch) not significantly different from normal control subjects for either temporal lobe, whereas the ratio NAA/Ch was decreased and the ratio NAA/Cr was highly increased in the hamartoma [55, 76].

Cerullo *et al.* recently reported evidence that gelastic seizures are accompanied by an abrupt sympathetic system activation. The authors speculate that this phenomenon is probably due to the «direct paroxysmal activation of limbic and paralimbic structures or other autonomic centres of the hypothalamus and medulla» [11]. These results strongly infer that, at least at the beginning of the disease, HH is directly responsible for seizure through proper epileptogenicity. These findings have been paralleled with those reported in focal cortical dysplasia which is also considered to be properly epileptogenic [7]. Similarly, epileptogenicity of cortical dysplasia has been demonstrated with reference to electro-cortico-graphic abnormalities of the lesion at the operation [53] and with regard to in vitro epileptogenicity of surgically excised lesions [41], ictal SPECT studies showing hyperperfusion in lesions themselves [34], and surgical failures when removal of the dysplasia was partial [51, 53].

The Effect of GKS on epileptic tissue is now well established

Our experience with mesial temporal lobe epilepsy (MTLE) constitutes a further rationale for treating epilepsy with GK. In 1993 we initiated a program dealing with the application of GK surgery for the treatment of MTLE without space occupying lesions (but with hippocampal sclerosis) [63, 66]. First results [64] suggested a high rate of efficacy (81%), absence of mortality and a very low rate of permanent neurological deficit (3 visual field deficits among 25 patients). This approach has also some disadvantages as opposed to microsurgical resection [60, 64]. Firstly, sufficient material is not yet available for final evaluation. Secondly, seizure cessation occurs with a delay of 6 to 21 months (median 10,5) and aura cessation with a delay of 9 to 22 months (median 15,5) [64]. Thirdly, image changes appearing on the MR [68] around 11 months (9–22) are generally completely asymptomatic but more rarely have been associated with headache, nausea, and vomiting which are rapidly resolved with steroids [64] .We promoted the idea [65] that the same efficacy regarding seizure could certainly be attained with lower doses, thus avoiding these transient image changes [65]. Our experience with Gamma Knife Surgery for lesions located in highly functional cortex associated with epilepsy also shows that epilepsy can resolve without destructive action and without any neurological deficit [60, 61]. Such clinical facts led us to speculate that it would perhaps be possible to modify an epileptogenic cortex sufficiently to be no longer epileptic while sparing its ability to assume its functional role. We demonstrated the existence of biochemical differential effects in an experimental model [65]. In this model the cholinergic system had reduced activity and amino excitatory acid levels were very much reduced in spite of preservation of the Gabaergic system as assumed through GAD and Gaba level stability [65]. The problem then was to identify the dosimetry parameters (what dose and what dose distribution, for a specific volume and location) in order to obtain a reproducible effect on seizure while sparing the underlying function and avoiding structural lesions. In this sense HH associated with epilepsy provides an excellent model if we accept the hypothesis that the epileptogenic zone is limited under these very special circumstances to the boundary of the lesion. In the retrospective study, while all patients were improved, 4 of them are currently seizure free (one case with only residual auras). These patients received the highest dose on the HH suggesting a dose related effect. Indeed, a dose of 17 Gy at the margin seems to be sufficient to cure a high percentage of patients when the epileptogenic zone is completely covered. However it is clear that with marginal doses under 13 Gy there is little chance of seizure cessation. In contrast to what was observed after radiosurgical treatment of MTLE [68], in this group of patients treated with smaller target volume and lower doses, none of our patients has experienced any kind of MR changes until now. This total absence of high T2 signal in the months following radiosurgery provides supplementary evidence of the possibility to induce an antiepileptic effect without necrosis [27].

Epilepsy associated with hypothalamic hamartoma often is severe refractory epilepsy with incapacitating behavioural abnormalities and cognitive decline. Recently a retrospective study has demonstrated the efficacy and low morbidity of Gamma Knife Surgery (GKS) in patients with hypothalamic hamartoma (HH) associated with severe epilepsy [59]. Since Arita's case report [4] and our series two papers have confirmed the efficacy and safety of radiosurgery [21, 80].

In order to address more cautiously the important issue of middle/long term safety and efficacy in this group – mainly children with catastrophic epilepsy – we have organized a multicenter prospective study controlled by an ethic committee and the health authorities.

We must underline that only very preliminary results are available concerning the prospective trial. Also in the literature, due to the rarety of this diagnosis, series reported have always been extremely small (from one to 5 cases) except the retrospective multicenter series of Palmini [52] aggregating 13 cases. Our series of 30 prospectively evaluated patients is unique. by the number of patients and the strict methodology of this evaluation.

Time course of events: when to evaluate and when to conclude failure?

The majority of patients have a similar time course of events. Delays in occurrence of these events differ from one individual to the other. The typical pattern comprises 5 periods spread over a minimum of two years. At first patients experience generally a quite immediate global improvement with reduced seizure frequency, and severity is usually associated with an improvement in behaviour. During the following months (more frequently from month 2 to month 6), frequency of seizures is back to the preoperative state. However, these seizures are generally shorter with less or no loss of contact. Fifty percent of the patients during this period predominantly have seizures with no objective signs, according to the family, but the patient still experiences the initial subjective part of seizures (auras). A decrease in drugs during this period can lead to the occurrence of a series of complex partial seizures or even generalized seizures (3 cases). In the second period, despite a constant number of seizures, other parameters start to improve. At that period background EEG and sleep normalize, behaviour improves, the capacity to gain new acquisition at school grows, the overall quality of live ameliorates. Then suddenly the third period sets in, which is marked by a peak of seizures with sometimes a large number of seizures in only a small number of days. Duration of this period is of some days or weeks, rarely more than a month. When this period is long, peaks of seizures generally have a lower amplitude. The fourth period is marked by seizures disappearing progressively. The fifth period is the consolidation period when the patient is completely seizure free. Interindividual variability exists mainly in the delay of onset and duration of these periods and in the amplitude of the clinical phenomenon described above. However, knowledge of this pattern obtained from typical patients is very helpful for the follow-up of more atypical patients in whom these milestones generally are present but more discrete and still of great value for situating the patient in the ongoing cure process.

Effects on precocious puberty: The mechanisms underlying such phenomenon remain unclear. Neurosecretory granules containing GnRH have been shown to be present in surgically removed hamartomas which correspond to heterotopic nervous tissue [14]. Commentz *et al.* have observed in a young girl with central precocious puberty and gelastic seizures due to a hypothalamic hamartoma melatonin plasma levels low for the chronological age but appropriate for the pubertal status, leading the author to suspect a causal relationship between lowered melatonin plasma levels and precocious puberty [13]. In the retrospective study three patients had precocious puberty. Among these two were treated too late to assess efficacy of radiosurgery on that condition. In the third patient radiosurgery performed at 6 years did not lead to subsidence of precocious puberty. In the prospective trial of the 20 patients experiencing PP only 2 were treated early enough to evaluate the influence of radiosurgery on that condition. GnRH analog treatment is supposed to be stopped at two years. A 2-year-follow-up is not yet available for these two patients. Surprisingly, in the Melbourne experience with microsurgical resection by transcallosal approach (S. Harvey, personal communication Montreal 2002), none of the precocious puberties was remedied by resection (10 patients of the series of 23 presented a PP). Several series have reported the efficacy of microsurgery to correct PP in patients without associated epilepsy and presenting with pedunculated HH [1, 75]. Cure was reported after complete microsurgical removal of HH [1, 35, 75] or sometimes after partial resection only [35]. Albright *et al.* in 1993 reported of a successful surgical series of 5 children with hypothalamic hamartoma (4 pediculate and 1 sessile) and precocious puberty [1]. Four of the 5 patients exhibited postoperative oculomotor palsy requiring eye-muscle surgery in one case (3 were transient). The morbidity rate for resecting hypothalamic hamartoma with precocious puberty as reported by Albright and Stewart can be lowered by a pterional approach [1, 2, 75]. In the past decade, gonadotropin-releasing hormone analogs (GnRHas) have also been used effectively to treat precocious puberty. In the Stewart series all patients treated with decapeptyl had complete suppression of their puberty [75]. Stewart, in 1998, compared medical (in 4 patients) and surgical treatment (in 2 patients) and recommended medical treatment due to the proven efficacy of GnRHa for suppression of puberty and reducing advancement of bone aging because in his experience surgery was not effective for completely reversing the signs of puberty [75]. Interestingly, disappearance of the lesion was reported in rare cases [26] with a super long-acting hormone releasing hormone analogue (TAP-144-SR). GK radiosurgery could be an interesting alternative treatment for precocious puberty but to our knowledge has never been reported in this indication. However, the proven efficacy of GnRHa in suppressing puberty and reducing advancement of bone aging has led the majority of authors to advise against surgery as initial management of central precocious puberty caused by HH [75].

Safety: according to our short/middle term experience is excellent. No adverse neurological, psychological or visual sequelae, no diabetes insipidus, no appetite stimulation or other endocrinological sequelae were observed. Long term risks must be discussed. The use of radiotherapy (fractionated low doses in a large volume) in patients with brain disease compatible with long survival (e.g. pituitary tumors) have led to the incidence of new benign tumor or even sometimes malignancy in a significant percentage of patients [9, 73]. Since 1957 thousands of patients have been treated with radiosurgery around the world (more than 300 000 only with gamma knife). The vast majority of these patients are young and have been treated for benign disease. If the risk of tumorgenesis with radiosurgery had been equivalent to the one of radiotherapy, we should observe today thousands of tumors induced by these treatments. Clearly such a risk has not shown with radiosurgery. It is of great importance to point out the fact that radiobiology of radiotherapy and radiosurgery are very much different. Today some rare cases of patients treated with radiosurgery have been reported experiencing several months or even years after the operation the development of a new malignant tumor close to the initial target of radiosurgery. A causality relationship between radiosurgery and the new tumor is unlikely in several of these cases and a matter of debate in several others. However, even if all these rare cases were accepted as related to radiosurgery, the risk should appear still very low. No doubt, even if there is a risk of developing several years after radiosurgery a radio-induced tumor, this risk is very low and far lower than the risk to die following microsurgery (1–2%). On the other hand, the epileptologic, neuropsychologic and psychosocial prognosis of these children is catastrophic and beyond comparison with the oncological risk of radiosurgery. However parents are systematically informed of this potential risk.

Specific difficulties of radiosurgery in HH

The two main difficulties are the close relation to surrounding critical structures (optic tract, chiasma and mammillary bodies) and the poor delineation of the upper part of the lesion, frequently undistinguishable from the surrounding hypothalamus. Hamartomas are supposed by definition to correspond to normal grey matter in an abnormal place. This implies that radiological interpretation of borders to distinguish hamartomas from the surrounding structures could be problematic and in fact, even with high quality MR, precise delineation of the HH is difficult [6]. However in certain cases (3 of 5), some radiological studies have described the presence of a rim of isointense signal with a hyperintense center on T2-weighted sequences [79]. According to our previous prospective trial a marginal dose of 17 Gy was delivered when volume and relationship to surrounding critical structures rendered it possible. In the retrospective series there is a very clear correlation between efficacy and dose [59]. The patients in the successful group had significantly ($p = 0{,}029$) higher doses at the margin (median 18,6 Gy) as compared to the «not seizure free» group (median 12,00 Gy). The marginal dose was greater than 17 Gy for all patients in the successful group. The strategy during the operation is to prioritize sparing of the surrounding critical structures which leads us to optimize the gradient of the dose fall-off by using different tricks (including shielding and multiisocentrism) and by lowering the energy delivered to the lesion in its boundaries adjacent to these critical structures.

Pertinence of our topological classification

Classically clinical presentation of HH depends on its anatomy [3, 15, 81]. This issue has been addressed by Valdueza [81], Debeinex [15] and Arita [3] in their personal series of 6, 19 and 11 cases, respectively. According to these authors, pedunculated HH attached to the floor of the third ventricle or suspended from the floor by a peduncle are associated with PP or asymptomatic. These lesions correspond to type I of Valdueza [81] or the "parahypothalamic type" of Arita [3]. Sessile HH called by Valdueza type II and by Arita the "intrahypothalamic type," are associated with seizures. In this type, the hamartoma involves or is enveloped by the hypothalamus and eventually distorts the third ventricle (Type IIB of Valdueza). According to Arita, two thirds of patients with the pedunculated type experience developmental delays, and half also exhibit precocious puberty. Generally, patients without neurological and psychiatric symptoms (PP or asymptomatic patient) had pedunculated lesions suspended from the floor of the third ventricle and patients with neurological symptoms (with or without PP) had sessile *hamartoma* located in the hypothalamus with extension to the interpeduncular cistern. Surprisingly, one of our patients (patient n°10 in Table 1) with a pediculated type (Fig. 5) presented a severe epilepsy and psychiatric aggressivity problems. It could be of importance to note that this patient had a XXY caryotype (Klinefelter syndrome). As underlined by Palmini, exact location of the lesion in relation to the interpeduncular fossa and the walls of the third ventricle correlated with the extent of excision, seizure control, and complication rate [52]. This rationale led us to classify more precisely the HH according to their topology and relying on the pertinent features correlating with clinical semiology prognosis and surgical strategies (see Fig. 1). Even if we are reporting an exceptional observation, type IV (pediculated) have generally no neurological symptoms (no epilepsy, no cognitive deterioration and no behavioural disturbances). They can present with precocious puberty or be free of any symptom [12].

Type I, II and III in a great number of cases may cause seizures, mental retardation behavioural abnormalities and precocious puberty. Type V are frequently found in patients with particularly severe presentation. In our experience indications are better reaffined relying on such a topological classification.

Table 1. *Preoperative parameters*

N°	Name	MS	Type	D	Age	Gel	PC	Gen	PP	Behaviour abnormalities	Cognitive impairment	VM def
1	J.B.	–	IV+III+	23,4	12	1,0	3,9	–	+	aut+++	low average	–
2	C.F.	+	III	21,4	13	0,2	7,0	10,4	+O	+Aut?	retarded+++	+
3	V.Z.A.	–	II	12,5	20	7,8	7,8	8	–B	inh/aut	normal	–
4	C.S.	–	III	13,5	16	0 ?	4,7	5,4	+	–inh/aut	normal	–
5	A.C.	–	III	14,3	3	0,1	0,1	–	+	–hyperk	normal	–
6	M.L.	–	II+IV	14,1	12	1,9	5,6	8,9	+O	–hyperk aggress	low	–
7	A.P.	–	II	15,7	8	0,2	4,7	–	+	–hyperk aggress	low average	–
8	Y.D.	–	III+I	17,5	20	7,6	1,4	1,6	+	+hyperk aggress++	retarded++	–
9	F.B.	–	IV+I	14,3	19	0,4	0,4	–	+	+aut? halluc	retarded++	–
10	D.A.	–	V	9,4	22	0,0	6,3	–	+	+aggre parox++	low	–
11	L.K.	–	III	11,7	11	0,5	5,7	5,7	+	+aggre predator	normal	–
12	L.M.	–	II	8,5	30	3,6	6,3	–	+	–aggre parox++	low average	–
13	H.M.	–	IV	9,4	31	19	19	26	+	anxiety inhibition–	normal	–
14	C.G.	–	II	10,3	17	0,0	4,5	14,5	+	–	normal	–
15	H.A.	–	II	13,3	30	0,0	11,9	–	–	hyperk aggr anx	normal	–
16	J.D.	–	IV+III	12,8	14	0,0	1,4	8,0	+	aggressivity+	retarded++++	–
17	M.S.	–	II	10,3	40	5,1	8,1	8,1	–	inh/aut	low average	+
18	P.M.	–	II	7,2	38	9,1	9,1	14,1	+	+aggres hallu neurol	low average	+
19	L.H.	+	I+II	10,4	16	?	?	?	+O	opp hyper aggre	retarded++++	–
20	P.D.	–	IV+III	23,1	12	0,4	0,1	1,7	+	+aggressivity	low average	
21	J.L.	–	IV+III	13,7	3	1,3	1,9	–	–	+hyperk aggress++	normal	–
22	E.B.	–	II	8,2	16	0	6,3	7,3	–	inh/aut depress	retarded++++	–
23	G.A.	–	III	12,5	6	5,0	8,0	–	–	inhibition	normal	–
24	S.M.	–	IV+III	25	6	0,1	3,6	–	+	–obsessiv aut	low average	+
25	T.N.	–	II	10	23	0,0	6,7	6,7	O–	–inhibition anxiety	low average	+
26	M.M.	–	II	8,4	16	0,1	7,8	7,8	+	opposant aggressive	retarded++	+
27	L.C.	–	II	9	29	0,0	0,0	15,6	+	–	normal	+
28	N.B.	+	III	9,2	17	1,0	6,4	6,4	–	+aggre hallu neurol postop	low average	–
29	E.P.	–	II+I	9,5	18	0,0	12,3	12,3	–	+hyperk aggress++	normal	–
30	K.H.	–	II+I	10,5	13	0,5	–	10,1		–aut	normal	+

A+ in the MS (microsurgery) column means the patient has previously been operated. For classification of the different topological kinds of hamartoma refer to Fig. 1. Age is the age at the time of radiosurgery. The following column (*Gel; PC; Gen*) indicate the age of onset (in years) of gelastic (*Gel*), partial complex (*PC*) and generalized (*Gen*) seizures. A minus (–) means that this kind of seizure have never been reported by the patient physicians or the family. A+ in the column PP means that the patient has presented a precocious puberty. Behaviour abnormalities and cognitive impairment were rated from + to ++++ (0 if absent). For behaviour abnormalities (*inh*) mean inhibition (*aggr*) mean aggression and (*hyp*) means hyperkinetic according to the proeminence of the kind of behavioural abnormalities. «Hall» means that episode of hallucination have been reported. A+ in the column «VM def» indicates that the neuropsychological testing have demonstrated the existence of mnesic deficit uniquely or predominantly on the verbal aspect

Extent of HH treatment or resection

We can speculate that an incomplete treatment increases the risk of failure to control epilepsy and/or associated behavioural abnormalities and cognitive decline. A recent perusal of the literature [40, 45–47, 81] and an analysis of the data from 25 cases treated surgically by several groups led to the conclusion that only patients treated by total or subtotal resection of the hamartoma could be seizure-free [78]. However, some data are not congruent with this dogma. First, for radiosurgery complete coverage of the HH did not appear to be mandatory since for two patients of the successful group in our retrospective study dose planning spared a significant part of the lesion. Similarly some authors recommend a resection "conservative" enough to avoid complications relying on their experience with successful partial removal [82]. In several series patients with only partial resection and seizure cessation are reported [55, 70, 82]. In the Melbourne series completeness of resection turned out to be not predictive of the probability for seizure cessation (A. Simon Harvey, Personal communication, Montreal, December 2001). In this series of 21 patients, resection was considered «near complete» (95–100%) in 62% (13/21) of the patients and partial (25–90%) in 38% (8/21). The authors explain the high rate of partial resection by the anterior attachment to the chiasm or infe-

Table 2. *Summary of the results of the main surgical techniques for treatment of HH associated to severe epilepsies*

Complications	Palmini polkey	Harvey	Delalande	Guthrie	Dubeau benabid	Pallini	Murphy	Regis
	Pterional	Transcallosal	Combined	Thermocoagulation	Deep stim	Callosotomy	VNS	GKS
Population	13	5/21	18	12	2	1	6	8/30
Hypernatremia > 150		/12 (0)		?				0
Diabetus insipidus	1		1/18 (0)	?				0
Somnolence		/7 (0)	?	?				0
Temperature instability		/5 (0)	?	?				1 (0)
III nerve unilateral palsy	4 (0)	/1 (0)	1/18 (0)	1/12 (0)				0
Thalamocapsular or Thalamic infarct	4	/2	1/18 (0)	0				0
Brainstem infarct	0	0/0	0	1/12 (1)				0
Hemiplegia			1/18 (1)	1				0
Hemiparesis			1/18 (0)	0				0
Meningitis			1/18 (0)	0				0
Hyperphagia +− obesity	1	/10 (5)	2/18 (0)	0	1/2			0
Low thyroxine		/6 (4)	?	?				0
Anxiety depression		/4 (3)	?	?				2
New short term memory deficit		/8 (3)	0	1/12 (0)				0
Infection				*	*			0
Hematom				**	**			0
Seizure cessation	15% (2/13)	40%/67%	56% (10/18)	(25%) 3/12	0%	0%	0%	50% 4/8
Seizure reduction > 90%	50%–77%	24%	44%				3/6	50% 4/8
No worthwhile improvement	31%–8%	5%	0%				3/6	0
Behaviour improvement	13/13					0	4/4	6/6
EEG improvement						0		5/5
Developmental Acceleration	4/13					0		3/8
Efficacy delay	no	no	no	no	y	no	y	y

* Frequent in larger series for other indications.

rior extension to the pontine level or a broad base on the lateral hypothalamus or a large HH distorting the 3rd ventricle. In spite of this high rate of partial resection via the transcallosal approach, these authors reach a rate of seizure cessation similar to the one reported in other microsurgical or radiosurgical series (66%). Also, results on seizures are not better in patients with complete resection. Convergingly using several contacts or electrodes in the same lesion, Kahane reported different independent "epileptogenic zones" inside the latter (without involvement of the other regions) and which could sometimes be distinguished by different clinical semiology (Kahane, personal communication 1999). Although GKS does not seem to be suitable when the lesion is large, «radiosurgical» disconnection can perhaps be envisaged by radiosurgically targeting only the superior part in the hypothalamus and/or the 3rd ventricle leaving untreated all lesion lower than the floor. As a matter of fact, only one of the two patients treated according to this strategy has sufficient evaluation for follow-up and is a failure. The second patient is a young girl, aged 12, operated by gamma knife 1 year ago. She experienced an initial seizure reduction then was back to the preoperative state concerning frequency with shorter and less severe seizures, clearly improved behaviour, and better performance at school noticed by the teachers. Even if it is too early to predict seizure cessation, supposed to occur in the following months, undoubtedly she is already very much improved. In both cases we recommended microsurgery as first intention but the parents after having been informed of the risks where scared and opted for radiosurgery.

Preoperative predictors of success?

In our retrospective study only treatment at an earlier stage, when epilepsy is not yet too severe, was related with a higher chance of seizure freedom following radiosurgery. In our retrospective study the successful group had significantly ($p = 0,03$) less gelastic seizures before radiosurgery (median 6 gelastic seizures/month) compared to the «not seizure free» group (median 45 gelastic seizures/month) [59]. Preoperatively the capacity to deliver optimized doses at the margin (which mean small type I and II or III HH) was a positive predictor. According to the Melbourne team, additionally to the low severity of the epilepsy (absence of «symptomatic generalized epilepsy» $p = 0,003$), the intellectual normality ($p = 0,006$) was also a positive predictor of a good outcome in terms of seizure freedom (S. Harvey, personal communication, Montreal 2001).

How does GKS compare to the different alternative strategies?

The possibility of curing associated epilepsy with a treatment limited to the HH was suggested in some studies. In 1969, Paillas was the first to demonstrate that improvement of seizure by surgical resection of HH without morbidity could be achieved [49].

Palmini aggregated the cases treated in Montreal (McGill), London (King's College) and Porto Allegre and reported a series of 13 HH with severe epilepsies treated by microsurgical resection [52]. This important work confirms the efficacy of surgery when orientated toward the HH. In this series, 3 out of 13 patients treated by microsurgical resection showed complete seizure cessation and seizure reduction was superior to 90% in 10 of these 13 patients. It is also noteworthy that removal of the HH, when complete, can suppress both kinds of seizures [81]. Unfortunately according to Valdueza [81], epilepsy in HH is observed only in medium/large sessile HH broadly attached to tuber cinereum or mamillary body [81]. Microsurgical resection in this critical area is related to a significant risk of occulomotor palsy, hemiparesis and visual field deficit, and a lot of epilepsy surgeons have therefore abandoned this approach [1, 2, 17, 40, 45–47, 72, 75, 81]. Palmini reports 4 thalamocapsular infarcts with contralateral hemiplegia subtotally recovered, a transient third nerve paresis in 4 patients, a central diabetes insipidus and a nonreversible hyperphagia [52].

The Melbourne team proposes to approach HH via a *transcallosal-interforniceal* route to the third ventricle. This team published in January 2001 a series of 5 cases operated by this route. Two of the patients were seizure free, two others very much improved. No permanent complications were reported except two appetite stimulations (one developing obesity). Some months later the Melbourne team (S. Harvey, Personal Communication, Montreal, December 2001) reported a series of 25 patients operated by the same route including 21 with sufficient follow-up for evaluation (FU = 3–52 months). Results were not so favorable as regards complications in this larger group but more favourable in terms of seizure cessation rate (67% instead of 40%). Resection was near complete (95–100%) in 13 of the 21 (62%). Some transient side effects were reported: hypernatremia (> 150) in 12 (57%), somnolence in 7 (30%), body temperature instability in 5 patients (24%), third nerve palsy in 1 patient. Permanent complications were also reported: thalamic infarct in two cases (one capsulo-thalamic), appetite stimulation in 10 cases (48%), permanent in 5 (24%), low thyroxin level in 6, permanent in 4 (19%), anxiety and depression in 4, permanent in 3, and short term memory deficit in 8 patients (38%), permanent in 3 (15%). In this group of 21 patients a sum of 38 transient complications and 18 permanent complications occurred. The more important concern, according to the author himself, is with memory complaints.

Delalande, due to an occurrence of severe complications after his first case, has switched to simple *disconnection*. When the clinical result is not satisfactory and the upper part of the lesion is mainly in the third ventricle, this author proposes a second step via an endoscopic approach to the 3rd ventricle. He reported (personal communication, Montreal, December 2001) a series of 18 patients with HH with a mean follow-up of 28 months. In this excellent series half the patients are in class I of Engel. The author reports some permanent severe complications with 1 hemiplegia, 1 secondary hemiparesis, 2 hyperphagia and some transient morbidity (1 meningitis, 1 diabetes insipidus). It is of importance to note that the majority of these complications have occurred after operation of the first cases. Other than the team using the transcallosal approach, the author reports no memory deficit and no other endocrine deficit. In contradiction to the other teams, Delalande observed a correlation between completeness of exclusion and result on seizures.

Some authors have proposed *stereotactic radio-*

frequency thermocoagulation lesioning of HH instead of direct microsurgical approach [32, 54]. Due to the irregular conformation and close proximity to the normal hypothalamus, mammilary bodies, and visual pathways, direct lesioning with a stereotactic probe carries a certain risk. Also the interface between HH and the normal hypothalamus may be unclear and perforating vessels "en passage" (e.g. thalamo perforate) may be possible. Guthrie (personal communication, Montreal, 2001) reports of 12 cases of thermocoagulation (mainly small lesions). Of 12 patients only 3 were seizure free which looks like less successful than microsurgery or radiosurgery. The author reports some transient complications (1 transient third nerve palsy, and a transient mnesic deficit) and a very severe in one patient (brainstem infarction). Additionally we know from the literature that a 1–2% risk of hemmorrhage is associated with all insertions of stereotactic probe in the brain. Finally according to the author, the main disadvantages of this technique are blindness of the probe pass, difficulty to impact the hamartoma, absence of control over the extent of the physical effect and theoretical requirement of multiple probe passes (implying an increment in risk) due to the complexity of shape and relationship to critical structures in the majority of cases.

Other authors proposed *stimulation of the HH* like the Grenoble team. The patient reported by this team was significantly improved after stimulation but the severity of the side effects (weight gain) led him to abandon this technique. Sadikot and Dubeau reported a patient they have implanted both in the anterior thalamus and the HH. Until now the clinical results don't seem to be more favorable.

Finally the *vagus nerve stimulation* has been described by Murphy *et al.* [44]. The authors reported results of a left vagus nerve stimulation in six children with HH and epilepsy. In this small group none were seizure free, 3 were improved and 3 not significantly improved. This experience indicates clearly that vagus nerve stimulation is a poorly effective therapy as compared to radiosurgery or microsurgery, where almost all patients are improved and more than 50% seizure free. This limitation in efficacy, the costs, the requirement for battery change every 4–5 years and the 3% risk of infection related to pacemaker implantation, in our opinion, must lead to consider vagus nerve stimulation only as second or third intention when radiosurgery and/or microsurgery have failed and/or are contraindicated. However, in such circumstances there are several arguments in favour of vagus nerve stimulation instead of callosotomy. Efficacy of *callosotomy* is even more limited [50] (Dubeau, personal communication, Montreal, 2001), surgical risk is higher, and impact on behaviour and psychiatric symptoms is very poor. On the opposite, in the paper of Murphy and coworkers [44], of 4 patients with severe autistic behaviour all 4 were dramatically improved by the intermittant stimulation (VNS).

Indications of radiosurgery in HH

Due to the influence of the timing of radiosurgery (or surgery) on the chance of seizure cessation and reversal of the epileptic encephalopathy, early surgical intervention is probably to be recommended in an attempt to minimize or prevent the cognitive and behavioural sequelae commonly seen with this epileptic syndrome.

Marked improvement of generalized seizures with resection of the HH despite depth electrode demonstration of apparent neocortical onset have been reported [28]. In as much as preoperative electro-clinical data and depth electrode recordings turn out to be inaccurate for predicting outcome regarding seizure cessation [10, 28] indications are at present mainly based on anatomical aspects in patients with severe drug-resistant epilepsies.

Small HH located inside the hypothalamus extending more or less in the third ventricle (stage I+II) or in the floor are certainly the best candidates for GKS. In this population the risk of microsurgical removal is likely to be potentially high. When the lesion is small and mainly in the third ventricle (Type II or II+I), radiosurgery is certainly the safer alternative. Even though the endoscopic and transcallosal approach have been proposed, the risks of short term memory worsening, endocrinological disturbance (hyperphagia with obesity, low tyroxine, sodium metabolism disturbance) and thalamic or thalamocapsular infarct have been reported also by the more enthousiastic and skillful neurosurgeons. If the lesion is small and sessile in the cistern (type III) gamma knife surgery can be recommended due to its safety and due to its capability to reach at the same time also the small associated part of the lesion in the hypothalamus itself frequently visible on the high resolution MR. If the lesion is of type III but too big for radiosurgey, a pterional approach is usually recommended. When the lesion is large or pediculate in the cistern, microsurgical removal or

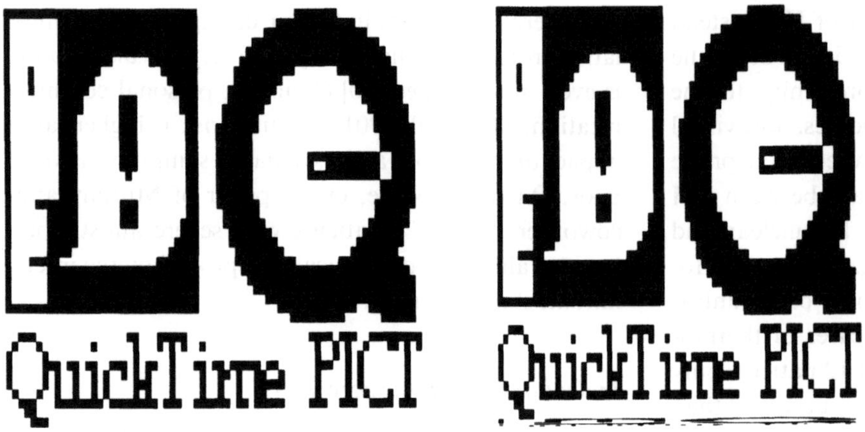

Fig. 3. Mixed type (Type I+III). This patient is presenting with a mixed type (III+II) of HH. The lesion is surrounding the mammilary body on the right and is posterior to fornices

disconnection must be discussed. Although GKS does not seem to be suitable when the lesion is large, «radiosurgical» disconnection can perhaps be envisaged (radiosurgery targetting only the superior part in the hypothalamus and/or the 3rd ventricle leaving untreated all the lesion lower than the floor). When microsurgical resection has left a small remnant in the third ventricle and a still active epilepsy, re-operation can be envisaged by GKS. For re-treatment after a first GKS procedure, the key point is to take into account the observed probability of seizure cessation depending on time (Fig. 4). Due to the existence of inter-individual variability (late responders) we recommend waiting for 36 months after first radiosurgery before proposing a second treatment. The excellent safety of gamma knife surgery and the history of successful results with retreatment are strong arguments to propose a second step radiosurgery in patients with only seizure reduction and a small HH. There are few doubts that gamma knife surgery is the least invasive surgery we can propose to these children with a similar efficacy. Contraindicated are big or giant lesions (stage IV) as well as patients with extremely severe psychiatric disorder. Indications of different neurosurgical approaches (radiosurgery, endoscopy, transcallosal, pterional resection or disconnection) appear complementary.

Reversal of the epileptic encephalopathy

In the literature, onset of epilepsy ranges from 1 day to 15 years (mean 2.8 years) [78]. Brief gelastic seizures or more rarely dacrystic seizures are generally the first ones to occur and are refractory to drug therapy [8, 28, 78]. During evolution other types of intractable seizures generally occur including complex partial seizures with or without secondary generalization and tonic or tonicoclonic generalized seizures. Seizures with fall are described in 50% of cases in patients aged more than 15 years. In addition, precocious puberty and progressive mental decline are commonly reported. Therefore, evolution of the disease is considered to be invariably unfavorable when several types of seizures, the worsening of EEG features (progressively marked by generalized discharges) and mental impairment occurs [78]. Deonna have aggregated the arguments suggesting that the acquired cognitive and behavioural symptoms result from a direct effect of the seizures [18]. These authors speculate that epilepsy location and its spread from the hypothalamus are responsible for the early neurobehavioural profile and combines features of a pervasive, developmental and attention deficit disorder. Interestingly, in our experience, reversal seems to start before complete cessation of seizures and looks more like correlated to the improvement of background EEG activity. Difazio *et al.* insisted on the precocity of the onset of specific clinical signs in neonatal cases and on the value of the SPECT [19]. EEG background is frequently disorganized by frequent interictal activity. During sleep normal organisation often is altered. These two electrical features are frequently normalized during the months following radiosurgery far before seizure cessation and concomitant with improvement in behaviour and cognitive functioning. SEEG recordings demonstrated the frequency of subclinical discharges in the HH and their

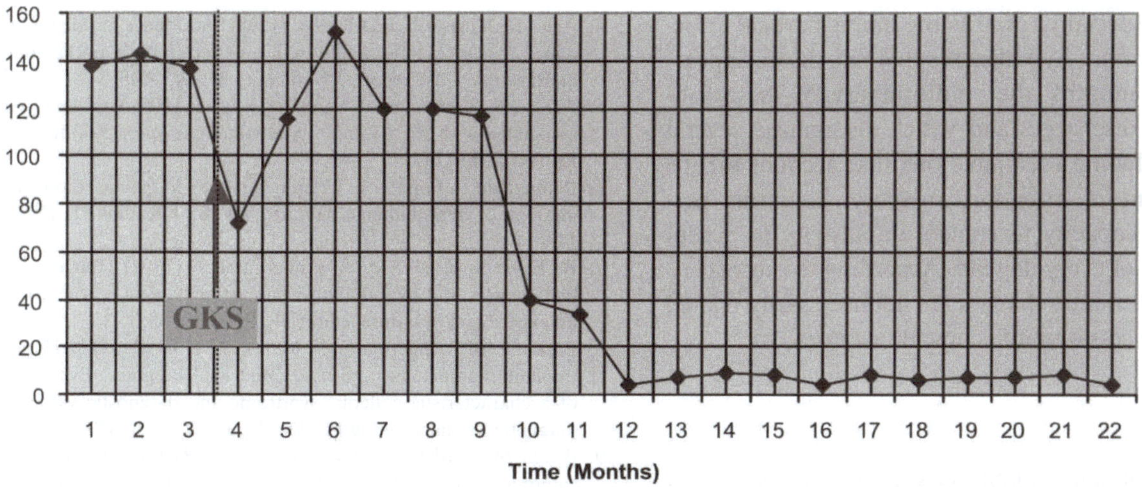

Fig. 4. Evolution of Global Seizure Frequency after Gamma Knife Surgery. After a discrete improvement in the following days or weeks, the seizure frequency is back to the preoperative status and even higher during some weeks, then around the 6th month the seizures start to decrease. A large variability exists between patients especially in the delay of these events; some patients are displaying these changes much later

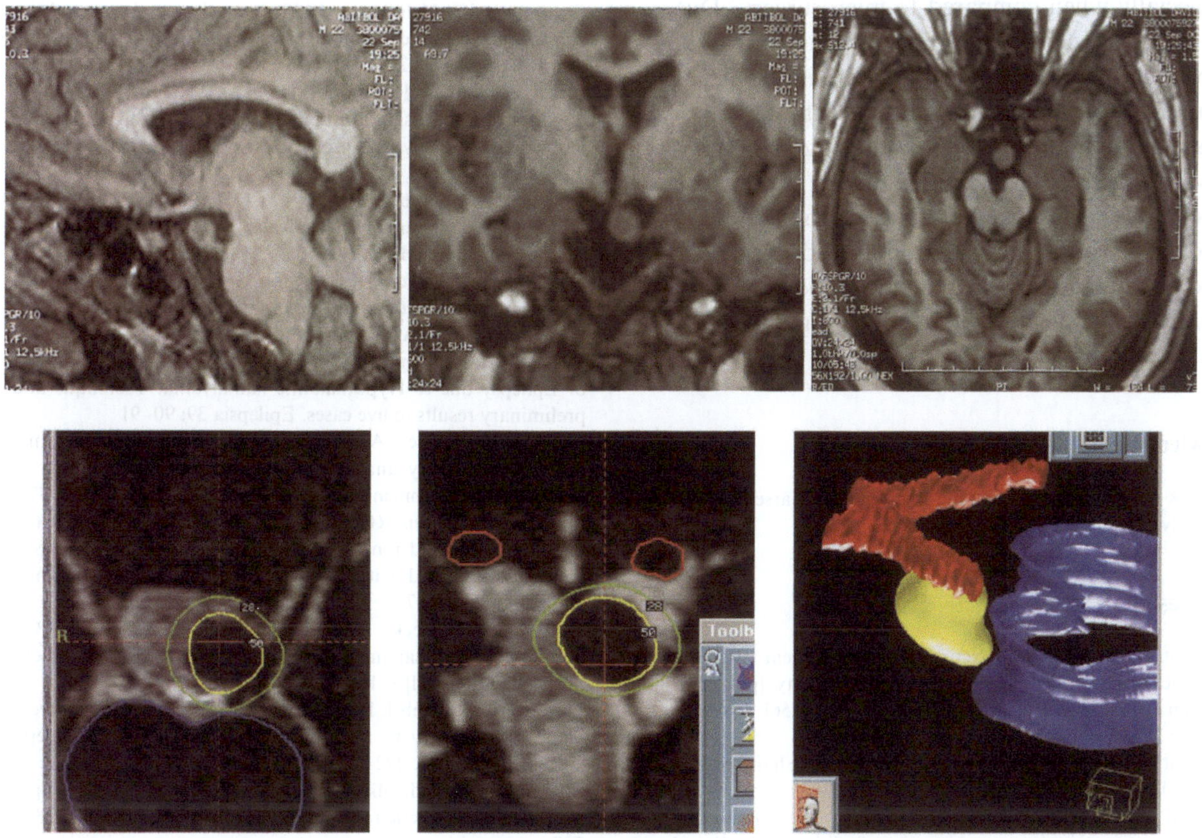

Fig. 5. MR imaging of case N°10. This patient is presenting with a pediculate type. In spite of this topological situation this patient had severe epilepsy and psychiatric aggressivity

spreading especially towards the limbic cortical structures. The author hypothezises that it is the disappearance some months after radiosurgery of these subcontinuous discharges and which disorganise several systems including the limbic one that account for the improvement of attention, memory, cognitive performances, capacity to control impulsivity to accept frustrations of every day life. According to our experience these dramatic changes are not necessarily related to complete cessation of «clinical» seizures.

Conclusion

The role of gamma knife surgery in epilepsy surgery has not yet been elucidated. Mesial temporal lobe epilepsies are treated efficiently and safely by microsurgical cortectomies. Consequently, radiosurgery is still considered experimental for this indication as long as no evidence for the superiority of gamma knife has been provided. The problem of HH is completely different. Radiosurgery can alleviate both the seizures and the behavioural and cognitive abnormalities of hypothalamic hamartomas and complications are very rare especially when compared to microsurgery. Due to the severity of clinical prognosis in the majority of these patients with HH and due to the invasivity of microsurgical resection, GKS can presently be envisaged as first intention for small/middle size HH associated with epilepsy as it may dramatically improve the future of these young patients. The role of secondary epileptogenesis or of cortical, widespread dysgenesis needs to be better evaluated and understood in order to identify the best indications and the best time point for Gamma Knife Surgery.

Acknowledgments

We thank the «Assistance Publique Hôpitaux de Marseille» who have actively supported this work.

References

1. Albright A, Lee P (1993) Neurosurgical treatment of hypothalamic hamartomas causing precocious puberty [published erratum appeared in J Neurosurg 1993 Jul;79(1):156]. J Neurosurg 78: 77–82
2. Albright A, Lee P (1998) Surgery for hypothalamic hamartomas [letter]. J Neurosurg 88: 353
3. Arita K, Ikawa F, Kurisu K *et al* (1999) The relationship between magnetic resonance imaging findings and clinical manifestations of hypothalamic hamartoma. J Neurosurg 91: 212–220
4. Arita K, Kurisu K, Iida K *et al* (1998) Subsidence of seizure induced by stereotactic radiation in a patient with hypothalamic hamartoma. Case report. J Neurosurg 89: 645–648
5. Arroyo S, Santamaria J, Sanmarti F *et al* (1997) Ictal laughter associated with paroxysmal hypothalamopituitary dysfunction. Epilepsia 38: 114–117
6. Beningfield S, Bonnici F, Cremin B (1988) Magnetic resonance imaging of hypothalamic hamartomas. Br J Radiol 61: 1177–1180
7. Berkovic S, Kuzniecky R, Andermann F (1997) Human epileptogenesis and hypothalamic hamartomas: new lessons from an experiment of nature [editorial]. Epilepsia 38: 1–3
8. Berkovic SF, Andermann F, Melanson D *et al* (1988) Hypothalamic hamartoma and associated ictal laughter. Evolution of a characteristic epileptic syndrome and diagnostic value of magnetic resonance imaging. Ann Neurol 23: 429–439
9. Brada M, Ford D, Ashley S *et al* (1992) Risk of second brain tumor after conservative radiotherapy for pituitary adenoma. Br Med J 304: 1343–1346
10. Cascino GD, Andermann F, Berkovic SF *et al* (1993) Gelastic seizures and hypothalamic hamartomas: evaluation of patients undergoing chronic intracranial EEG monitoring and outcome of surgical treatment. Neurology 43: 747–750
11. Cerullo A, Tinuper P, Provini F *et al* (1998) Autonomic and hormonal ictal changes in gelastic seizures from hypothalamic hamartomas. Electroencephalogr Clin Neurophysiol 107: 317–322
12. Cheng K, Sawamura Y, Yamauchi T *et al* (1993) Asymptomatic large hypothalamic hamartoma associated with polydactyly in an adult. Neurosurgery 32: 458–460; discussion 460
13. Commentz JC, Helmke K (1995) Precocious puberty and decreased melatonin secretion due to a hypothalamic hamartoma. Horm Res 44: 271–275
14. Culler FL, James HE, Simon ML *et al* (1985) Identification of gonadotropin-releasing hormone in neurons of a hypothalamic hamartoma in a boy with precocious puberty. Neurosurgery 17: 408–412
15. Debeneix C, Bourgeois M, Trivin C *et al* (2001) Hypothalamic hamartoma: comparison of clinical presentation and magnetic resonance images. Horm Res 56: 12–18
16. Degerblad M, Rähn T, Bergstrand G *et al* (1986) Long-term results of stereotactic radiosurgery to the pituitary gland in Cushing's disease. Acta Endocrinol 112: 310–314
17. Delalande O, Fohlen M, Jalin C *et al* (1998) Surgical treatment of Epilepsy due to Hypothalamic hamartoma: Technique and preliminary results in five cases. Epilepsia 39: 90–91
18. Deonna T, Ziegler AL (2000) Hypothalamic hamartoma, precocious puberty and gelastic seizures: a special model of "epileptic" developmental disorder. Epileptic Disord 2: 33–37
19. DiFazio MP, Davis RG (2000) Utility of early single photon emission computed tomography (SPECT) in neonatal gelastic epilepsy associated with hypothalamic hamartoma. J Child Neurol 15: 414–417
20. Donley D, Kuzniecky R, Mountz J *et al* (1994) Ictal SPECT findings in hypothalamic hamartoma and epilepsy (Abstract). Epilepsia 35 [Suppl] 8: 146
21. Dunoyer C, Ragheb J, Resnick T *et al* (2002) The use of stereotactic radiosurgery to treat intractable childhood partial epilepsy. Epilepsia 43: 292–300
22. Flickinger J, Kondziolka D, Lunsford L (1998) Clinical applications of stereotactic radiosurgery. Cancer Treat Res 93: 283–297
23. Flickinger JC, Kondziolka D, Lunsford LD (1998) Radiosurgery management of brain metastasis from systemic cancer.

In: Lunsford LD, Kondziolka D, Flickinger JC (eds) Progress in neurological surgery: gamma knife brain surgery. Karger, Basel, pp 145–159
24. Frattali CM, Liow K, Craig GH *et al* (2001) Cognitive deficits in children with gelastic seizures and hypothalamic hamartoma. Neurology 57: 43–46
25. Grob J, Regis J, Laurans R *et al* (1998) Radiosurgery without whole brain radiotherapy in melanoma brain metastases. Eur J Cancer 34: 1187–1192
26. Harada K, Yoshida J, Wakabayashi T *et al* (1995) A super long-acting LH-RH analogue induces regression of hypothalamic hamartoma associated with precocious puberty. Acta Neurochir (Wien) 137: 102–105
27. Hayashi M, Bartolomei F, Rey M *et al* (2002) MR changes after gamma knife radiosurgery for mesial temporal lobe epilepsy: an evidence for the efficacy of subnecrotic doses. In: Kondziolka D (ed) Radiosurgery. Karger, Basel, pp 192–202
28. Kahane P, Munari C, Minotti L *et al* (1997) Role of the hypothalamic hamartoma in the genesis of gelastic and dacrystic seizures. In: Tuxhorn I, Holthausen H, Boenigk H (eds) Pediatric epilepsy syndromes and their surgical treatment. John Libbey, London, pp 447–461
29. Kahane P, Tassi L, Hoffmann D *et al* (1994) Crises dacrystiques et hamartome hypothalamique : à propos d'une observation vidéo-stéréo-EEG. Epilepsies 6: 259–279
30. Kondziolka D, Lunsford L, McLaughlin M *et al* (1998) Long-term outcomes after radiosurgery for acoustic neuromas [see comments]. N Engl J Med 339: 1426–1433
31. Kondziolka D, Niranjan A, Lunsford L *et al* (1999) Stereotactic radiosurgery for meningiomas. Neurosurg Clin N Am 10: 317–325
32. Kuzniecky R, Guthrie B, Mountz J *et al* (1997) Intrinsic epileptogenesis of hypothalamic hamartomas in gelastic epilepsy. Ann Neurol 42: 60–67
33. Kuzniecky R, Guthrie B, Mountz J *et al* (1995) Hypothalamic hamartomas and gelastc seizures: evidence for subcortical seizure generation by ictal SPECT and cerebral stimulation. Epilepsia 36 [Suppl] 3: 266
34. Kuzniecky R, Mountz J, Wheatley G *et al* (1993) Ictal Single Photon emission computed tomography demonstrates localized epileptogenesis in cortical dysplasia. Ann Neurol 34: 627–631
35. Kyuma Y, Kato E, Sekido K *et al* (1985) Hypothalamic hamartoma successfully treated by operation. Case report. J Neurosurg 62: 288–290
36. Laws E, Vance M (1999) Radiosurgery for pituitary tumors and craniopharyngiomas. Neurosurg Clin N Am 10: 327–336
37. Leksell L (1951) The stereotaxic method and radiosurgery of the brain. Acta Chir Scand 102: 316–319
38. Leksell L (1971) Stereotaxis and radiosurgery. An operative system. In: Thomas CC (ed) Springfield
39. Lunsford LD (1990) Stereotactic radiosurgery of intracranial arteriovenous malformations. Neurosurgery update. Mc Graw-Hill, New York, pp 175–185
40. Machado HR, Hoffmann HJ, Hwang PA (1991) Gelastic seizures treated by resection of a hypothalamic hamartoma. Child's Nervous System 7: 462–465
41. Mattia O, Olivier A, Avoli M (1995) Seizure-like discharges recorded in human dysplastic neocortex maintained in vitro. Neurology 45: 1391–1395
42. Mori Y, Kondziolka D, Flickinger J *et al* (1998) Stereotactic radiosurgery for brain metastasis from renal cell carcinoma [see comments]. Cancer 83: 344–353
43. Munari C, Kahane P, Francione S *et al* (1995) Role of the hypothalamic hamartoma in the genesis of gelastic fits (a video-stereo-EEG study). Electroencephalogr Clin Neurophysiol 95: 154–160
44. Murphy JV, Wheless JW, Schmoll CM (2000) Left vagal nerve stimulation in six patients with hypothalamic hamartomas. Pediatr Neurol 23: 167–168
45. Nishio S, Fujiwara S, Aiko Y *et al* (1989) Hypothalamic hamartoma. Report of two cases. J Neurosurg 70: 640–645
46. Nishio S, Morioka T, Fukui M *et al* (1994) Surgical treatment of intractable seizures due to hypothalamic hamartoma. Epilepsia 35: 514–519
47. Nishio S, Shigeto H, Fukui M (1993) Hypothalamic hamartoma: the role of surgery. Neurosurg Rev 16: 157–160
48. Norén G (1996) Gamma knife radiosurgery for acoustic neurinomas. In: Gildenberg PL, Tasker RR (eds) Textbook of stereotactic and functional neurosurgery. Mc Graw-Hill, New York, pp 835–844
49. Paillas JE, Roger G, Toga M *et al* (1969) Hamarthome de l'hypothalamus. Rev Neurol 120: 177–194
50. Pallini R, Bozzini V, Colicchio G *et al* (1993) Callosotomy for generalized seizures associated with hypothalamic hamartoma. Neurol Res 15: 139–141
51. Palmini A, Andermann F, Olivier A (1991) Focal neuronal migration disorders and intractable partial epilepsy: results of surgical treatment. Ann Neurol 30: 750–757
52. Palmini A, Chandler C, Andermann F *et al* (2002) Resection of the lesion in patients with hypothalamic hamartomas and catastrophic epilepsy. Neurology 58: 1338–1347
53. Palmini A, Gambardella A, Andermann F (1995) Intrinsic epileptogenicity of human dysplastic cortex as suggested by corticography and surgical results. Ann Neurol 37: 476–487
54. Parrent AG (1999) Stereotactic radiofrequency ablation for the treatment of gelastic seizures associated with hypothalamic hamartoma. Case report. J Neurosurg 91: 881–884
55. Pascual-Castroviejo I, Moneo JH, Viano J *et al* (2000) [Hypothalamic hamartomas: control of seizures after partial removal in one case]. Rev Neurol 31: 119–122
56. Plouin P, Ponsot G, Dulac O *et al* (1983) Hamartomes hypothalamiques et crises de rire. Rev. EEG Neurophysiol 13: 312–316
57. Pollock BE, Kondziolka D, Lunsford LD *et al* (1994) Stereotactic radiosurgery for pituitary adenomas: imaging, visual and endocrine results. Acta Neurochir (Wien) 62: 33–38
58. Prasad D, Steiner M, Steiner L (2000) Gamma surgery for vestibular schwannoma [see comments]. J Neurosurg 92: 745–759
59. Regis J, Bartolomei F, de Toffol B *et al* (2000) Gamma knife surgery for epilepsy related to hypothalamic hamartomas. Neurosurgery 47: 1343–1351; discussion 1351–1342
60. Regis J, Bartolomei F, Hayashi M *et al* (2000) The role of gamma knife surgery in the treatment of severe epilepsies. Epileptic Disord 2: 113–122
61. Régis j, Bartolomei F, Kida Y *et al* (2000) Radiosurgery of Epilepsy Associated with Cavernous Malformation: Retrospective study in 49 patients. Neurosurgery 47: 1091–1097
62. Regis J, Bartolomei F, Metellus P *et al* (1999) Radiosurgery for trigeminal neuralgia and epilepsy. Neurosurg Clin N Am 10: 359–377
63. Régis J, Bartolomei F, Rey M *et al* (1999) Gamma knife surgery for mesial temporal lobe epilepsy. Epilepsia 40: 1551–1556
64. Regis J, Bartolomei F, Rey M *et al* (2000) Gamma knife surgery for mesial temporal lobe epilepsy. J Neurosurg 93 [Suppl] 3: 141–146
65. Régis J, Kerkerian-Legoff L, Rey M *et al* (1996) First biochemical evidence of differential functional effects following gamma knife surgery. Stereotact Funct Neurosurg 66: 29–38

66. Régis J, Peragut J, Rey M *et al* (1994) First selective amygdalo-hippocampic radiosurgery for mesial temporal lobe epilepsy. Stereotact and Functional Neurosurg 64 [Suppl] 1: 191–201
67. Régis J, Peragut JC, Rey M *et al* (1994) First selective amygdalohippocampic radiosurgery for mesial temporal lobe epilepsy. Stereotact Funct Neurosurg 64: 191–201
68. Regis J, Semah F, Bryan R *et al* (1999) Early and delayed MR and PET changes after selective temporomesial radiosurgery in mesial temporal lobe epilepsy. AJNR Am J Neuroradiol 20: 213–216
69. Roche PH, Régis J, Dufour H *et al* (2000) Gamma knife Radiosurgery in the management of cavernous sinus meningiomas. J Neurosurg 93: 68–73
70. Rosenfeld JV, Harvey AS, Wrennall J *et al* (2001) Transcallosal resection of hypothalamic hamartomas, with control of seizures, in children with gelastic epilepsy. Neurosurgery 48: 108–118
71. Rutigliano MJ, Lunsford LD, Kondziolka D *et al* (1995) The cost effectiveness of stereotactic radiosurgery versus surgical resection in the treatment of solitary metastatic brain tumors. Neurosurgery 37: 445–455
72. Sato M, Ushio Y, Arita N *et al* (1985) Hypothalamic hamartoma: report of two cases. Neurosurgery 16: 198–206
73. Simmons NE, Laws E (1998) Gliomas Occurence after sellar Irradiation: case report and review. Neurosurgery 42: 172–178
74. Steiner L, Lindquist C, Adler J *et al* (1992) Clinical outcome of radiosurgery for cerebral arteriovenous malformations. J Neurosurg 77: 1–8
75. Stewart L, Steinbok P, Daaboul J (1998) Role of surgical resection in the treatment of hypothalamic hamartomas causing precocious puberty. Report of six cases. J Neurosurg 88: 340–345
76. Tasch E, Cendes F, Li LM *et al* (1998) Hypothalamic hamartomas and gelastic epilepsy: a spectroscopic study. Neurology 51: 1046–1050
77. Tassi L, Quarato P, Francione S (1995) Chronological relationships between ictal laughing and smiling and intralesional discharges: stereo-EEG study of a patient with gelastic epilepsy and hypothalamic hamartoma. Epilepsia 36: 239–240
78. Tassinari CA, Riguzzi P, Rizzi R *et al* (1997) Gelastic seizures. In: Tuxhorn I, Holthausen H, Boenigk H (eds) Current problems in epilepsy. John Libbey, London, pp 429–446
79. Turjman F, Xavier J, Froment J *et al* (1996) Late MR follow-up of hypothalamic hamartomas. Childs Nerv Syst 12: 63–68
80. Unger F, Schrottner O, Haselsberger K *et al* (2000) Gamma knife radiosurgery for hypothalamic hamartomas in patients with medically intractable epilepsy and precocious puberty. Report of two cases. J Neurosurg 92: 726–731
81. Valdueza J, Cristante L, Dammann O *et al* (1994) Hypothalamic hamartomas: with special reference to gelastic epilepsy and surgery. Neurosurgery 34: 949–958; discussion 958
82. Watanabe T, Enomoto T, Uemura K *et al* (1998) [Gelastic seizures treated by partial resection of a hypothalamic hamartoma]. No Shinkei Geka 26: 923–928
83. Weissenberger AA, Dell ML, Liow K *et al* (2001) Aggression and psychiatric comorbidity in children with hypothalamic hamartomas and their unaffected siblings. J Am Acad Child Adolesc Psychiatry 40: 696–703

Correspondence: Dr. J. Régis, Service de Neurochirurgie Fonctionnelle et Stéréotaxique, C.H.U. La Timone, 264 rue Saint Pierre, 13385 Marseille, Cedex 05, France. e-mail: jregis@ap-hm.fr

Acta Neurochir (2004) [Suppl] 91: 51–54

Gamma knife radiosurgery for nonfunctioning pituitary adenomas

A. Muacevic[1], E. Uhl[2], and B. Wowra[1]

[1] German Gamma Knife Center Munich, Ludwig-Maximilians University, Munich, Germany
[2] Department of Neurosurgery, Ludwig-Maximilians University, Munich, Germany

Summary

The efficacy of gamma knife radiosurgery (GKS) for nonfunctioning pituitary adenomas (NPAs) has been assessed. Sixty patients with NPA were treated by GKS. Complete neurological and endocrinological follow-up information was available for 51 patients. Follow-up examinations included stereotactic magnetic resonance imaging for sequential measurements of the NPA volume. The median dose to the tumor margin was 16.5 Gy (range 11–20 Gy). The mean prescription isodose was 50% (range 45–75%). All patients underwent surgery for NPA before GKS. Fractionated radiotherapy was not applied. Median follow up after GKS was 21.7 months. Actuarial recurrence-free survival was 95% after three years with respect to a single GKS and 100% for patients who underwent repeated GKS. No neurological side effects were detected. Two patients developed new partial pituitary insufficiency after radiosurgery. Postoperative GKS for residual or recurrent small fragments of NPAs is an effective and safe treatment option. The follow-up examination for NPAs should include tumor volumetric analysis.

Keywords: Radiosurgery; gamma knife; non-functioning pituitary adenoma; volumetric analysis.

Introduction

Pituitary adenomas represent about 14% of all intracranial tumors. In the majority of cases these tumors are associated with pathological hormone secretion. Approximately one third of them are nonfunctioning pituitary adenomas (NPA) [22]. At presentation they are mostly large extrasellar macroadenomas causing neurological symptoms by compression of surrounding structures. In these tumors, reduction of the tumor volume is the major aim of therapy which is done by surgical debulking in most cases. However, many tumors may not be completely resected because they are in the proximity to critical structures or invade the cavernous sinus. Because residual adenomatous tissue is associated with a higher risk of tumor recurrence, radiosurgery may be indicated after surgery if the lesion volume is small and the distance of the adenoma surface to the optic pathway is sufficiently broad to enable a safe procedure. To define the treatment effects of radiosurgery for these small lesions, precise volumetric analysis of the tumors would be superior to the crude approximation of tumor size measurement by determining tumor diameters. Magnetic resonance imaging provides the possibility of measuring discrete tissue volumes. Therefore, the purpose of this study was to assess the efficacy of GKS for NPAs including a protocol of sequential tumor volumetric analysis based on stereotactic MR imaging follow-up studies.

Material and methods

Sixty patients (median age: 50 years, range: 21–77 years) with nonfunctioning pituitary adenomas were treated with outpatient GKS between October 1994 and April 2004 at our institution. Conventional fractionated radiotherapy was not applied. All patients had undergone prior resection of their NPA. The median dose to the tumor margin was 16.5 Gy (range 11–20 Gy). The mean prescription isodose was 50% (range 45–75%). Follow-up stereotactic MR imaging was performed by placing the patient's head into the localizer box of the Leksell stereotactic system, which was coupled to the Leksell stereotactic base frame. In contrast to the treatment procedure, the frame was not rigidly fixed to the patient's skull for the follow-up examinations. Identical MR imaging sequences, however, were used for both the follow-up studies and the treatment planning. A coronal turbo-flash sequence with injection of the contrast medium during imaging was used to identify adenoma tissue and the pituitary gland, respectively. In addition, a three-dimensional volume scan was obtained to determine adenoma volume. The slice thickness of this sequence was 1.5 mm and the matrix was 256 * 256, delivering a voxel size of 0.98 mm^2 in the x–y plane. Hence, the volume of the image voxels was 1.5 mm^3. An MR imager (Expert 1.0 tesla; Siemens, Erlangen, Germany) was used for all examinations [16]. To check for MR image distortions, all patients were also examined with computer tomography (HigQ; Siemens, Erlangen, Germany) for treatment planning but not for follow-up examination. The first follow-up examination after GKS was performed after

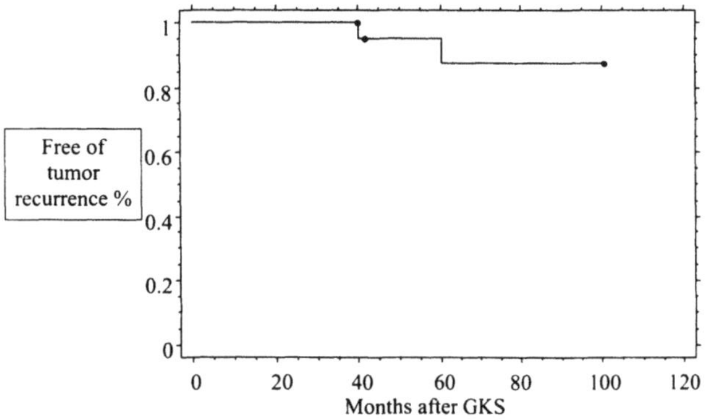

Fig. 1. Is showing the actuarial recurrence free survival for patients with non-functioning pituitary adenomas treated by gamma knife radiosurgery. 95% of the patients had a recurrence free survival of 3 years. *GKS* Gamma Knife Surgery

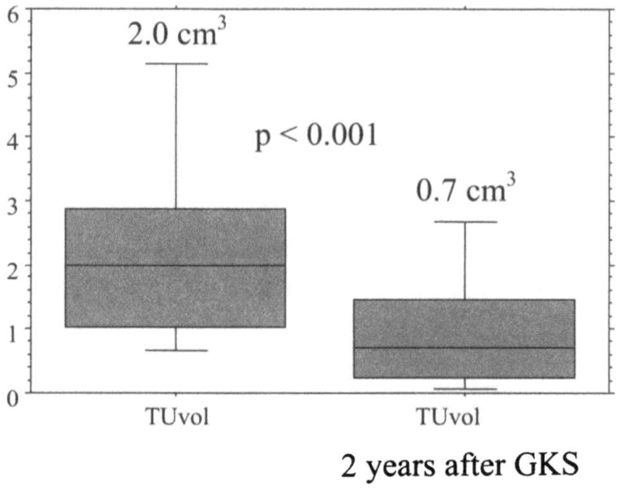

Fig. 2. Is illustrating the reduction of tumor volume (TUvol) after gamma knife radiosurgery. There was a significant tumor volume reduction from initial 2 cm^3 before GKS to 0.7 cm^3 two years after GKS

6 months. Thereafter, patient follow-up examinations were done once every year. These follow-p examinations included neurological. ophthalmological, and endocrinological tests. Radiation-induced pituitary insufficiency was defined as a requirement for new hormonal replacement medication after GKS or as a requirement for a dose increase in preexisting hormone therapy.

Results

The median follow-up period was 21.7 months (range 4.9–100.6 months), 51 complete examinations were performed after GKS in 60 NPA patients. Patients underwent one to five follow-up examinations (median two). A new ophthalmological or focal neurological deficit was not recorded. In one patient a small asymptomatic tumor hemorrhage was observed on MR imaging. Two patients developed partial pituitary insufficiency after radiosurgery. One of these patients required de novo hormonal substitution therapy. In three individuals GKS was performed twice because of tumor recurrence. The actuarial long-term recurrence-free survival was 95% after three years and 90% after 5 years with respect to a single radiosurgical procedure (Fig. 1) and 100% if repeated GKS was included. Tumor recurrences were correlated with a lower maximum dose ($Dmax = 21 \pm 5$ Gy vs $Dmax = 30 \pm 5$ Gy; $p = 0.02$). The initial median tumor volume of 2 cm^3 (range 0.4–9.1 cm^3) decreased to 0.7 cm^3 (range 0.0–6.7 cm^3) after 2 years ($p < 0.001$) (Fig. 2).

Discussion

After surgical debulking, fractionated radiotherapy reduces the likelihood of tumor regrowth in patients with residual non-functioning pituitary adenomas [1, 3, 5, 13, 20, 37]. For fractionated radiotherapy, a dose–effect relationship has been determined [7, 19]. Decreased tumor control was found to be associated with increasing field size, which corresponded with large macroadenomas [6, 9, 32]. However, fractionated radiotherapy has well-known side effects such as radiation induced hypopituitarism which may develop several years after radiotherapy for NPAs [4, 21, 26]. Hypopituitarism following fractionated radiotherapy develops in 50 to 60% of treated patients using surgery and radiotherapy [32]. It is important to know that patients with hypopituitarism have an almost doubled risk of death (predominantly from vascular and respiratory disease) as compared with healthy volunteers [33]. Using gamma knife radiosurgery, the dose to the radiosensitive tissues such as the hypothalamus and the pituitary stalk can in theory be kept much lower in comparison with the doses delivered by radiotherapy. This could be confirmed with the the low incidence of hypopituitarism after radiosurgery in the current study and is also in line with the findings in other radiosurgical series for pituitary adenomas [8, 10, 11, 14, 15, 18, 23, 28, 32].

The recurrence rate of NPAs is moderate with 6% after surgery alone [13] and 3 to 9% after combined treatment [1, 5, 34]. In the current study, a similar high tumor control rate was confirmed. The actuarial recurrence-free survival was 95% after 3 years with respect to a single GKS treatment for NPAs. Similar results have been reported by other authors for nonfunctioning pituitary adenomas [8, 10, 11, 14, 17, 18, 23, 28, 32].

Fractionated radiotherapy harbors a certain risk of developing second cancers and radionecrosis of nervous tissue [2, 29]. Therefore, restricting the radiation dose prescribed to these tumors is reasonable and reduces the risk of side effects. There are, however, limitations to radiosurgery. The relationship between the tumor and the visual pathways must be consistent with delivering a therapeutic dose to the tumor while not giving a potentially toxic dose to these pathways. Moreover, the adenoma target has to be clearly visible on the MR image. The latter is crucial when addressing the issue of tumor control after radiosurgery. In most instances residual adenoma is restricted to small fragments located in surgically inaccessible sites, such as the cavernous sinus [10]. Tumor volumetric analysis for pituitary adenoms, also referred to as tumor volume mapping, has to be taken into account. There are different methods available for tumor volumetric analysis [12, 24, 25, 27, 30, 31, 36]. A simple method is the one previously described by our group [35]. Follow-up studies require no rigid fixation of the stereotactic frame and are acceptable for the patient. The drawback of this procedure for the patient, however, is the need to return to the treatment center for follow-up examinations.

Conclusions

The low complication rate, the low radiation exposure to surrounding normal nervous tissue and the possibility of a dedicated volumetric follow-up analysis makes gamma knife radiosurgery highly attractive for residual nonfunctioning pituitary adenomas and should be applied whenever possible.

References

1. Brada M, Rajan B, Traish D *et al* (1993) The long-term efficacy of conservative surgery and radiotherapy in the control of pituitary adenomas. Clin Endocrinol (Oxf) 38: 571–578
2. Breen P, Flickinger JC, Kondziolka D *et al* (1998) Radiotherapy for nonfunctional pituitary adenoma: analysis of long-term tumor control. J Neurosurg 89: 933–938
3. Comtois R, Beauregard H, Somma M *et al* (1991) The clinical and endocrine outcome to transsphenoidal microsurgery of nonsecreting pituitary adenomas. Cancer 68: 860–866
4. Constine LS, Woolf PD, Cann D *et al* (1993) Hypothalamic-pituitary dysfunction after radiation for brain tumors. N Engl J Med 328: 87–94
5. Ebersold MJ, Quast LM, Laws ER Jr *et al* (1986) Long-term results in transsphenoidal removal of nonfunctioning pituitary adenomas. J Neurosurg 64: 713–719
6. Flickinger JC, Nelson PB, Martinez AJ *et al* (1989) Radiotherapy of nonfunctional adenomas of the pituitary gland. Results with long-term follow-up. Cancer 63: 2409–2414
7. Grigsby PW, Stokes S, Marks JE *et al* (1988) Prognostic factors and results of radiotherapy alone in the management of pituitary adenomas. Int J Radiat Oncol Biol Phys 15: 1103–1110
8. Hayashi M, Izawa M, Hiyama H *et al* (1999) Gamma knife radiosurgery for pituitary adenomas. Stereotact Funct Neurosurg 72: 111–118
9. Hughes MN, Llamas KJ, Yelland ME *et al* (1993) Pituitary adenomas: long-term results for radiotherapy alone and post-operative radiotherapy. Int J Radiat Oncol Biol Phys 27: 1035–1043
10. Ikeda H, Jokura H, Yoshimoto T (1998) Gamma knife radiosurgery for pituitary adenomas: usefulness of combined transsphenoidal and gamma knife radiosurgery for adenomas invading the cavernous sinus. Radiat Oncol Investig 6: 26–34
11. Izawa M, Hayashi M, Nakaya K *et al* (2000) Gamma knife radiosurgery for pituitary adenomas. J Neurosurg [Suppl] 3(93): 19–22
12. Kuroiwa T, Hirai T, Ohta T (1999) Meningioma followed up for radiological findings before and after radiosurgery: case report. Minim Invasive Neurosurg 42: 44–46
13. Lillehei KO, Kirschman DL, Kleinschmidt-DeMasters BK *et al* (1998) Reassessment of the role of radiation therapy in the treatment of endocrine-inactive pituitary macroadenomas. Neurosurgery 43: 432–439
14. Lim YL, Leem W, Kim TS *et al* (1998) Four years' experiences in the treatment of pituitary adenomas with gamma knife radiosurgery. Stereotact Funct Neurosurg 70: 95–109
15. Losa M, Valle M, Mortini P *et al* (2004) Gamma knife surgery for treatment of residual nonfonctioning pituitary adenomas after surgical debulking. J Neurosurg 100: 438–444
16. Mack A, Czempiel H, Kreiner HJ *et al* (2002) Quality assurance in stereotactic space. A system test for verifying the accuracy of aim in radiosurgery. Med Phys 29: 561–568
17. Marks LB (1993) Conventional fractionated radiation therapy vs. radiosurgery for selected benign intracranial lesions (arteriovenous malformations, pituitary adenomas, and acoustic neuromas). J Neurooncol 17: 223–230
18. Martinez R, Bravo G, Burzaco J *et al* (1998) Pituitary tumors and gamma knife surgery. Clinical experience with more than two years of follow-up. Stereotact Funct Neurosurg 70: 110–118
19. McCollough WM, Marcus RB Jr, Rhoton AL Jr *et al* (1991) Longterm follow-up of radiotherapy for pituitary adenoma: the absence of late recurrence after greater than or equal to 4500 cGy. Int J Radiat Oncol Biol Phys 21: 607–614
20. McCord MW, Buatti JM, Fennell EM *et al* (1997) Radiotherapy for pituitary adenoma: long-term outcome and sequelae. Int J Radiat Oncol Biol Phys 39: 437–444
21. Mechanick JI, Hochberg FH, LaRocque A (1986) Hypothalamic dysfunction following whole-brain irradiation. J Neurosurg 65: 490–494
22. Milker-Zabel S, Debus J, Thilmann C *et al* (2001) Fractionated stereotactically guided radiotherapy and radiosurgery in the treatment of functional and nonfunctional adenomas of the pituitary gland. Int J Radiat Oncol Biol Phys 50: 1279–1286
23. Mokry M, Ramschak-Schwarzer S, Simbrunner J *et al* (1999) A six year experience with the postoperative radiosurgical management of pituitary adenomas. Stereotact Funct Neurosurg 72: 88–100

24. Niemczyk K, Vaneecloo FM, Lemaitre L *et al* (1999) The growth of acoustic neuromas in volumetric radiologic assessment. Am J Otol 20: 244–248
25. Novotny J Jr, Novotny J, Vymazal J *et al* (1999) Assessment of the accuracy of volume determination using stereotactic magnetic resonance imaging. In: Kondziolka D (ed) Radiosurgery, vol. 3. Karger, Basel, 2000, pp 107–116
26. Pai HH, Thornton A, Katznelson L *et al* (2001) Hypothalamic/pituitary function following high-dose conformal radiotherapy to the base of skull: demonstration of a dose-effect relationship using dose-volume histogram analysis. Int J Radiat Oncol Biol Phys 49: 1079–1092
27. Peterson AM, Meltzer CC, Evanson EJ *et al* (1999) MR imaging response of brain metastases after gamma knife stereotactic radiosurgery. Radiology 211: 807–814
28. Pollock BE, Kondziolka D, Lunsford LD *et al* (1994) Stereotactic radiosurgery for pituitary adenomas: imaging, visual and endocrine results. Acta Neurochir (Wien) [Suppl] 62: 33–38
29. Popovic V, Damjanovic S, Micic D *et al* (1998) Increased incidence of neoplasia in patients with pituitary adenomas. The Pituitary Study Group. Clin Endocrinol (Oxf) 49: 441–445
30. Prasad D, Steiner M, Steiner L (2000) Gamma surgery for vestibular schwannoma. J Neurosurg 92: 745–759
31. Scheib SG, Gianolini S, Haller D *et al* (2000) VOLUMESERIES: a software tool for target volume follow-up studies with computerized tomography and magnetic resonance imaging. Technical note. J Neurosurg [Suppl] 3(93): 203–207
32. Shin M, Kurita H, Sasaki T *et al* (2000) Stereotactic radiosurgery for pituitary adenoma invading the cavernous sinus. J Neurosurg [Suppl] 3(93): 2–5
33. Tomlinson JW, Holden N, Hill RK *et al* (2001) Association between premature mortality and hypopituitarism: west midlands prospective hypopituitary study group. Lancet 357: 425–431
34. Tsang RW, Brierley JD, Panzarella T *et al* (1994) Radiation therapy for pituitary adenoma: treatment outcome and prognostic factors. Int J Radiat Oncol Biol Phys 30: 557–565
35. Wowra B, Stummer W (2002) Efficacy of gamma knife radiosurgery for nonfunctioning pituitary adenomas: a quantitative follow up with magnetic resonance imaging-based volumetric analysis. J Neurosurg 97 [Suppl] 5: 429–432
36. Yu CP, Cheung JY, Leung S *et al* (2000) Sequential volume mapping for confirmation of negative growth in vestibular schwannomas treated by gamma knife radiosurgery. J Neurosurg [Suppl] 3(93): 82–89
37. Zierhut D, Flentje M, Adolph J *et al* (1995) External radiotherapy of pituitary adenomas. Int J Radiat Oncol Biol Phys 33: 307–314

Correspondence: Alexander Muacevic, M.D., German Gamma Knife Center, Ingolstädterstr. 166, 80939 Munich, Germany. e-mail: Alexander.Muacevic@med.uni-muenchen.de

Acta Neurochir (2004) [Suppl] 91: 55–63

Gamma knife radiosurgery for cerebral arteriovenous malformations

A. A. Kemeny, M. W. R. Radatz, J. G. Rowe, L. Walton, and **A. Hampshire**

National Centre for Stereotactic Radiosurgery, Sheffield, UK

Summary

Since its introduction, gamma knife radiosurgery has become an important treatment modality for cerebral arteriovenous malformations. This paper is a brief overview of the technique used, of the clinical results achieved and of the experience gained in Sheffield.

Keywords: Cerebral arteriovenous malformation; stereotactic radiosurgery; gamma knife; multidisciplinary treatment.

Introduction

The introduction of stereotactic radiosurgery was initially received with scepticism in many circles, however, since that time the technique has found its way into the neurosurgical armamentarium in centres around the world. This was the result of the efforts of a small, enthusiastic and inventive group of neurosurgeons who, working with Lars Leksell, boldly tested the device on a wide range of indications. It is part of neurosurgical "folklore" that stereotactic radiosurgery in general and gamma knife surgery in particular was introduced primarily for functional indications. Indeed, the first prototype Gamma Unit was optimised for functional treatments by having slit-shaped collimators, whereas from the second prototype in 1975 onwards the collimators were round, making it more suitable for larger targets.

The first cerebral arteriovenous malformation treated with the gamma knife was reported by Steiner and Backlund in 1970 [25]. The importance of radiosurgery in the management of cerebral arteriovenous malformations was quickly realised when the first few pioneering treatments resulted in success. Early presentations and publications by Ladislau Steiner showed that, with the combination of foresight and perhaps some luck, the most useful paradigms had been established [26]. With later modifications and improvements in the technique that further enhanced the utility and efficacy of the method, AVM radiosurgery has proved to be one of the great "success stories" of modern neurosurgery.

The gamma knife unit in Sheffield was established in 1985 as a clinical research facility. Initially there was a specific emphasis placed on treating benign conditions rather than palliating malignant ones and the research programme concentrated on AVMs. Since then the Unit has become increasingly a clinical workhorse, indications and case mix have diversified and to date over 5700 patients have been treated. Reflecting the early vascular specialisation over 3000 of these patients have had AVMs. This paper is a brief overview of the techniques used, and of the clinical results and experience that has been achieved.

Material and methods

Patients

Between September 1985 and December 2003, 3096 patients were treated for an AVM. More than 90% of treatments were performed under local anaesthetic, although 211 cases, mainly paediatric patients, have been treated under general anaesthesia, and we routinely advise this for children under 12 years of age. Sex distribution was approximately equal (1636 male, 1460 female). Mean age at treatments was 36 years (range 1–75, median 35 years).

A haemorrhage was the principal presenting symptom (1918 patients, 62%). 327 patients (10%) presented with fits, although a further 705 developed seizures after a bleed or other presentation. 851 patients presented with other neurological deficits or symptoms e.g. with headaches possibly related to the AVM, or indeed were incidental findings.

At the time of the referral for radiosurgery 558 had motor, 277 sensory, 185 cerebellar and 196 visual deficits either as a result of haemorrhage or previous treatments. Previous treatments included microsurgery in 646, endovascular treatment in 400 and both in 143. In the last decade the proportion of previous treatments has changed: in recent years about 65–70% were primary treatments.

There was a predilection of eloquent deep-seated lesions in our material (430 were in the thalamus or basal ganglia, 83 in the brain stem) although interestingly there does not appear to be a referral bias dictated by hemispheric dominance. The mean nidus size was 4.9 cm^3 (SD 6.9). Four hundred and sixty were larger than 10 cm^3 in volume. A detailed retrospective analysis of the early cases is underway but the most recent cases have Spetzler Martin Grade I in 6.8%, Grade II in 29.1%, Grade III in 50.2%, Grade IV in 13.7% and Grade V in 0.2%.

Radiation technique

Stereotactic radiosurgery was carried out using the gamma knife. We had a model RBS (Nucletec, Switzerland) installed in 1985. This was replaced with a Gamma Knife Model C (Elekta, Sweden) in 2001. This update has resulted in some minor technical changes in the way we plan targets. The underlying principles of gamma knife radiosurgery however remain the same.

Radiosurgical planning was carried out between 1985 and 1992 using a locally modified KULA program, and from 1992 with GammaPlan (Elekta, Sweden). The complexity of planning has increased over the years from single field treatments in the initial years progressing to a median number of 6, and maximum of 22 in 2003. The imaging for radiosurgery planning started with cut sheet film subtraction angiography. This has been replaced with distortion corrected digital subtraction angiography co-registered with T2 and proton density stereotactic MRI.

We consider 25 Gy as being the standard dose prescribed to the AVM margin, and reflecting this, this is the median dose prescribed in our material. We consider a 2.5 Gy reduction for large lesions, if the AVM is eloquently sited, if the patient is young (age below 16 years) or if he/she had previous radiotherapy or radiosurgery. In practice we are reluctant to reduce the dose below 17.5 Gy for fear of compromising of the efficacy of the treatment and if the AVM were large and/or eloquently sited to permit such a dose we would decline to treat the case.

Follow up protocol

In the initial years CT scan was performed at 6 monthly intervals. As subclinical radiological changes around the nidus did not require treatment and symptomatic cases were scanned in any case, this practice was discontinued in the late 1980s. Subtraction angiography was carried out annually in the first 52 cases, but subsequently only at two years after treatment. In subtotally occluded cases the angiography is repeated at three and four years. Our current protocol is to carry out MRI/MRA and MRDSA [2, 17], at two years and if no nidus is demonstrated angiography is performed to confirm the obliteration. If there is persistent nidus on MRI scanning further imaging is deferred until 3–4 years after the treatment and second treatments scheduled after four years.

Results

A retrospective update of the database and its analysis is underway. For the purpose of this manuscript the interim analysis of a smaller subset was chosen, from the calendar year of 1994. Of 163 consecutive AVM patients, data remained incomplete in 41: thirteen returned abroad and were not contactable and twenty-eight patients from Great Britain had no angiographic endpoint. Twenty-one of the latter denied complications but refused follow-up investigations. One died without post mortem examination of unknown cause. We had no information on 6. Of the 22 UK patients with some clinical information one had temporary monoparesis and one rebled without ill effects. We had full data on 122 patients.

The treatment was successful in 83 cases: they had no residual early filling vein on follow up angiography although in 12 there was a faint mark of vascularity at the site of the nidus (Fig. 1). For 3 patients this was their second treatment. For 10 cases it took until the 4 year angiogram to achieve occlusion. A substantial subset of successful cases were of high Spetzler Martin grade (Fig. 2): 36 Grade III, 3 Grade IV and 2 Grade V. The latter two are particularly interesting: they were large elongated right fronto-temporo-parietal lesions, successfully treated without complications with 20 Gy minimum dose. The seizures worsened in 2 needing increased medication. There were 4 complications: 3 had temporary visual field deficit and one had hemiparesis which only incompletely resolved.

Substantial reduction but with residual shunt was the result in 25 cases. These were on the whole larger lesions: the mean AVM volume was 7.3 cm^3. This limited their radiation dose (21 ± 3.1 Gy, several as low as 15 Gy). Of the 25, 16 were re-treated with the gamma knife at a later stage, 13 successfully. One was embolised and the rest refused treatment. In this group two suffered hemiparesis and one dysphasia, the latter resolving without residual.

Very little size reduction was achieved in 14 cases, 11 of which were Spetzler Grade III or above. Two bled since the treatment, one of these being fatal. There were two neurological complications. None had further radiosurgery (it being the policy of our unit not to re-treat if the first response is minimal). However, 2 of the 14 had surgery later and 3 were embolised.

The results did depend on previous treatments. Both embolised and previously operated cases did worse than those treated primarily with gamma knife but only the former comparison achieved a level of significance ($p = 0.017$). The main factor in outcome prediction was size and Spetzler-Martin grade (Fig. 3). The near uniform dose selection in this material did not permit demonstration of a dose-dependent obliteration rate.

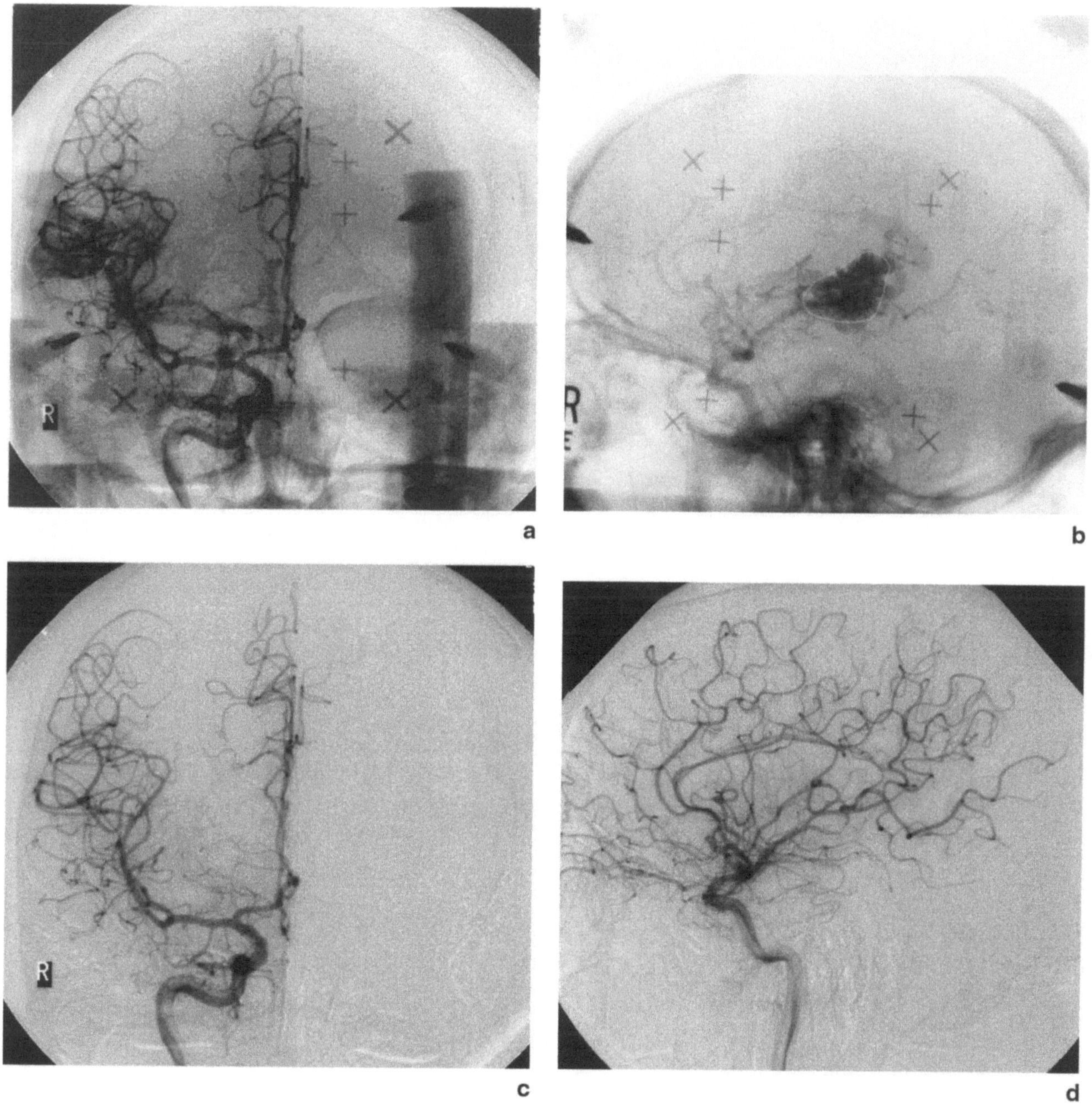

Fig. 1. Thrombo-obliteration response of an AVM 2 years after stereotactic radiosurgery with the gamma knife. 20 Gy peripheral ("minimum") dose used. (a) PA view at treatment, (b) lateral view at treatment, (c) PA view at 2 years, (d) lateral view at 2 years

In summary, safe obliteration was achieved in 83 of 122 cases (68%), rising to 81% if the later second gamma knife treatment was taken into consideration. Nine of the 122 (7.4%) had neurological complications, but only 5 (4.1%) permanent. In addition, there were 3 non-fatal bleeds. There was a ten-year mortality of 2/163 (1.2%), though only one case (0.6%) was confirmed to be caused by an AVM bleed and none due to the treatment.

Discussion

Once diagnosed, every patient harbouring an AVM has to consider one of four treatment strategies: observation, surgery, embolisation and radiosurgery.

Observation is an important management option. However, the natural history of cerebral AVMs is not precisely known. The range of reported annual incidence of haemorrhage is between 1%–5%. The predis-

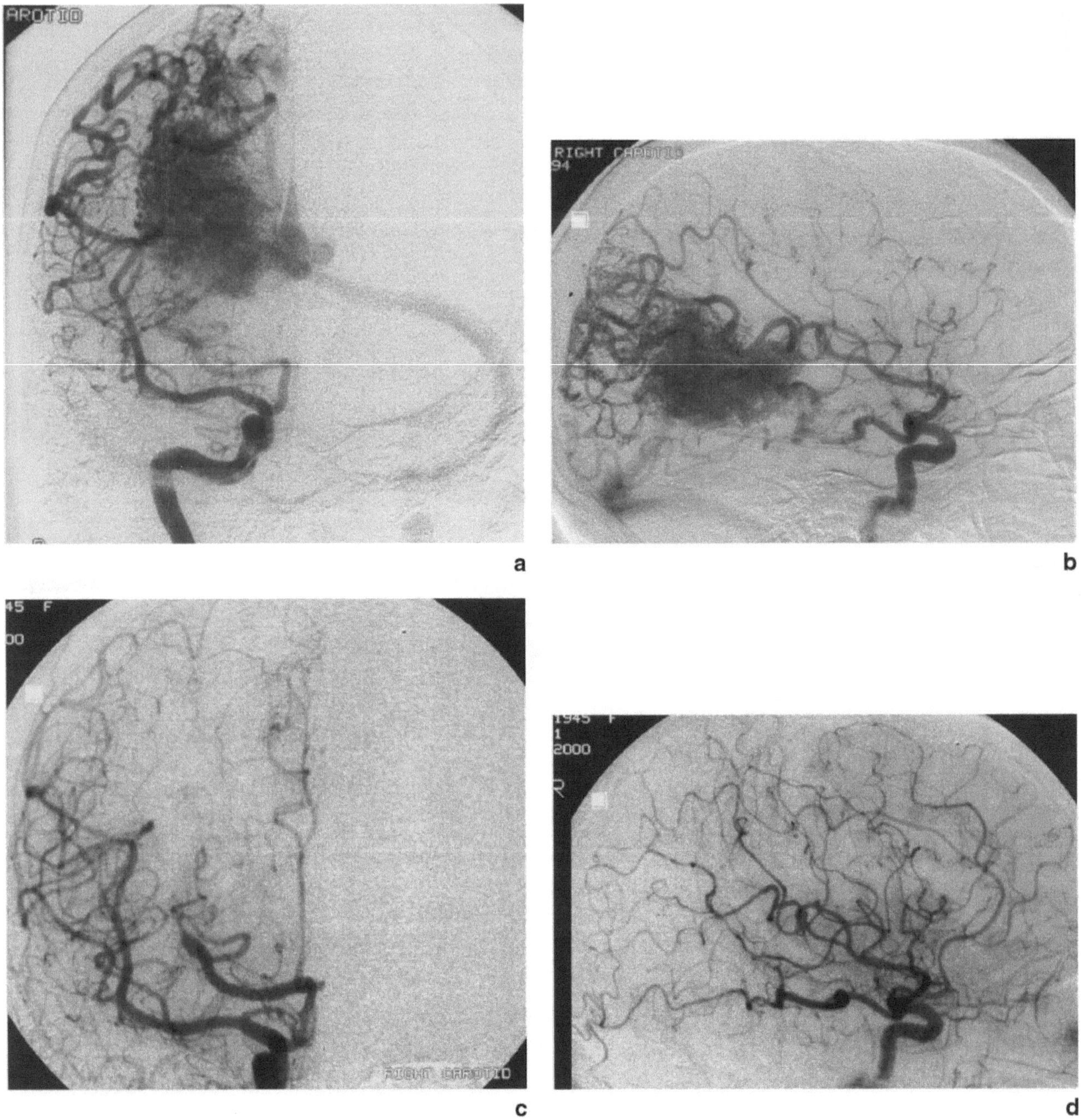

Fig. 2. Large AVM successfully treated with a single gamma knife treatment. (a) PA view at treatment, (b) lateral view at treatment, (c) PA view at 2 years, (d) lateral view at 2 years

posing factors for such a haemorrhage are also debated [14]. In particular, the role of nidus size is controversial: there are studies showing both that smaller or larger AVMs have higher risk for rupture, and some even concluded that the risk was independent of size. Previous haemorrhage was found by some to increase the risk in the first year whereas others found no such link. The annual risk of haemorrhage seems to increase with age but of course the cumulative lifetime risk for a young person is higher than that in the older age group. Small venous outflow and the presence of associated aneurysms probably increase the risk. These factors have to be carefully considered before observation is chosen.

Surgery has the advantage of offering an instant cure. Although a world apart from the heroic under-

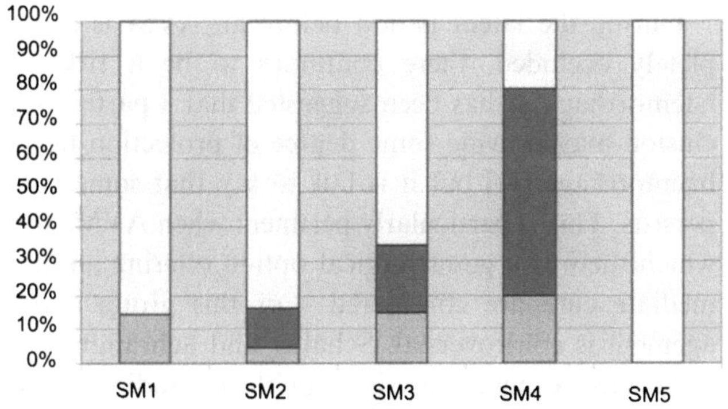

Fig. 3. Radiosurgical thrombo-obliteration is dependent on Spetzler-Martin grade which in turn is largely dependent on the size of the nidus. Legends: Occl = total occlusion, no early filling vein demonstrated. Subst = substantial reduction in nidus size but early vein persists. Min = minimal (less than 25%) reduction in nidus size. □ occl; ■ subst; □ min

takings of Olivecrona in the 1930s and aided by the microsurgical techniques introduced by Yaşargil in the 1970s, open surgery for cerebral AVMs remained a considerable challenge, carrying operative risks. These risks have been quantified using the Spetzler Martin grading system. The expected difficulties for the surgeon and the risks for patients often justify considering a non-invasive technique.

Embolisation is useful only for a subset of patients, depending on the angio-architecture of the nidus. Although the technology has evolved over the years, it is clear that endovascular interventions also carry their risks and have their limitations. A detailed analysis is of course beyond the scope of this paper.

Radiosurgery is the topic of this article. Some of the considerations surrounding this technique are discussed below.

Patient selection

Patient selection for radiosurgery is related to but not the same as selection of the ideal treatment plan for the individual patient. The ideal case for radiosurgical treatment is a patient with a small compact and non-eloquently placed AVM. Of course the same would also be the ideal case for open surgery, the only difference being that a surgeon would favour a lesion on the surface with superficial venous drainage, whereas for radiosurgery a deep-seated lesion is an easier target to treat than a superficial one.

At the start of the radiosurgical program in Sheffield in 1985 these ideal cases were selected. Since that time increasingly larger malformations have also been accepted. It rapidly became apparent that one could not deliver the same high dose in a single fraction to a large volume as one can to a smaller volume. To avoid complications the radiation dose to periphery of a large target, the so-called minimum dose, has to be reduced. Although a maximum diameter of 3 cm is usually accepted, volume is a more important factor. It is easy to appreciate that a "sausage shaped" elongated AVM has a smaller volume, and thus it is more suitable, than a spherical lesion of the same maximum diameter.

The shape of the lesion has other implications in patient selection. Comparing lesions of the same volume it is much easier to plan treatment for a smooth globular shape than for a craggy irregular lesion. The planning software, GammaPlan allows such intricate plans but both planning and treatment delivery are more time-consuming. The other shape-related factor is the proportion of different diameters. Considering the extreme, a thin flat nidus, e.g. a dural malformation does not lend itself to planning when the plan means overlapping several near-spherical treatment fields to match the shape.

It is also important that the margins of the nidus should be readily identifiable. Diffuse malformations are not only difficult to delineate but, because within the outlined target volume some normal parenchyma may be included, the risk of treatment may be higher. The same effect hinders treatment of post embolisation cases, though including axial imaging to some extent overcomes these difficulties.

When a treatment plan is formulated for an individual patient, many individual factors have to be considered, including those related to the patient in general, the lesion in particular and even those defined by the available facilities (Table 1).

Preoperative imaging

The above considerations make it clear that high quality digital subtraction angiography is necessary for assessment of the case for suitability. This allows for the assessment of the nidus and it also allows assessment of the speed of flow. The most important aspect of this assessment is the identification of a possible direct fistula. Direct arteriovenous fistulae do not respond well to radiosurgery whereas they are usually easily treatable with endovascular techniques. In some

Table 1. *Factors considered in management decisions for cerebral AVMs*

Radiological factors	
- Draining veins (deep or superficial)	surgical factors
- Size	
- Site (eloquence)	
- Diffuseness of nidus	radiosurgical factors
- Shape of nidus	
- Angio-architecture, nidal aneurysm	embolisation factors
Patient factors	
- Clinical state	
- Presentation	
History of bleed	
Epilepsy	
Steal phenomenon	
- Age (lifetime risk if untreated)	
- Patient's expectations and wishes	
Departmental factors	
- Skills available (surgery, endovascular, radiosurgery)	

cases supra-selective angiography is necessary to explore this possibility.

Over the recent years an increasing number of patients are referred following MRI or CT scanning without the benefit of DSA. In some cases (e.g. those with a small compact nidus) this may be acceptable but most centres would expect exploration of the angio-architecture using DSA before a treatment plan is formulated.

The relationship of the AVM nidus to eloquent structures is explored using MRI. Lesions in or near the speech areas or motor cortex could benefit from such an approach. In order to gain the maximum benefit from these scans, fusion of them to the planning imaging (see below) may be required.

The process

When exposed to ionising radiation, arteriovenous malformations undergo a slow histological change. Over the months following radiation, myofibroblasts form in the vessel adventitia, and under the endothelium collagen and hyaline deposits are laid down [16, 23, 27, 28]. As a result the targeted vessels progressively occlude. It may very well be that the slow time course of these changes contributes to the safety of the method by altering the haemodynamics only gradually. A speedier reaction could be achieved by higher radiation doses but the incidence of permanent untoward neurological sequelae may then rise.

During the latent period before an AVM is completely occluded, there continues to be a risk of haemorrhage. It has been suggested that a partial occlusion may provide some degree of protection from haemorrhage [11] but it is fair to say that some risk persists. This is particularly pertinent when AVMs for which there is a good surgical option offering an immediate cure are considered. For this group management is controversial. Schaller and Schramm [29] performed a meta-analysis of published radiosurgery results for low surgical risk AVMs. In this excellent surgical series the outcome appeared better than radiosurgery, if the analysis of the latter included the statistical risk of haemorrhage during the latent period. However, the rate of new or worsened deficits after surgery was 27.4% – a figure many times that of gamma knife-treated patients.

It has been suggested that the presence of the lesion during the latent period may cause anxiety or depression. The psychological effects of the delayed radiosurgical obliteration have been investigated in a study. There was no quality-of-life effect of the delay [13].

Management of large and eloquent AVMs is less controversial: no treatment modality claims high rate of success in isolation. Lesions with high Spetzler-Martin Grade have a high neurosurgical risk. Surgery has to be cautious leading to not infrequent post-surgical remnants particularly with AVMs located in the thalamus, basal ganglia and brainstem [15]. Surgery for these deeply placed AVMs carries a high surgical risk [18]. The supportive role of endovascular treatment has been identified over the past decade. With the introduction of acrylic glue instead of particle emboli, and subsequently Onyx, durable and sequential reduction of the volume can be achieved. Whereas a few decades ago this was invariably followed by excision of the remnant, increasingly a radiosurgical treatment follows embolisation. However, at all stages of sequential treatment of these difficult malformations, all three active interventions should be considered [1, 24]. Sequential treatments may involve several endovascular treatments followed by one or more radiosurgical interventions and in some the last remnant, particularly if superficial, is removed surgically.

In our own material there was a significantly worse post-radiosurgical occlusion rate in pre-embolised AVMs compared with primarily treated or indeed surgically reduced malformations and the same has been observed by others [20]. The reasons for this effect may be multiple. First, there may be a selection bias. Second, there is a poorer definition of the nidus margin as a result of embolisation and the presence of the agent used and this may result in suboptimal planning. Third, there may occur a recanalisation of the embolised part which was not demonstrable on angiography at the time of treatment. Whether the use of new materials e.g. Onyx will prevent these effects remains to be seen.

Some authors presented treatment of these large AVMs with sequential radiosurgery without utilising other modalities [19, 22]. The "traditional" scenario was that after a standard radiosurgical treatment one waited for the 2–3 or even 4 years to demonstrate the full effect of the first treatment before the next intervention was carried out on the remnant. For a large malformation one may apply a different approach. One could treat the whole lesion with a small number of fractions, though fully fractionated treatment has been largely unsuccessful in the past. Perhaps a smaller number of fractions may allow safe delivery of a therapeutic dose without compromising efficacy. A third alternative is to treat a different part of the large nidus each time, leaving only a few months between treatment. Good results have been reported with such segmental radiosurgery. With two or more radiosurgical interventions, but particularly with short interval between the treatments, it is important to take into account the previous treatments with their precise dosimetry when the next irradiation is planned [22].

Complications

Though the aim is obliteration of the malformation, it must be achieved with the minimum morbidity. Untoward events may be merely radiological or clinically relevant. On radiological level, Flickinger *et al.* [5] found that 30% of AVM patients had MRI changes adjacent to or within the irradiated volume at a median of 8 months after radiosurgery. These early changes are caused by a combination of altered perilesional blood flow [21], the rising of transluminal pressure as the nidus gradually obliterates and the blood brain barrier disruption with transudation of plasma proteins.

What is more important is any symptomatic change rather than any radiological one. In a multi-centre AVM study, 8% of patients developed neurological sequelae after radiosurgery [6]. Symptoms included focal neurological deficit, cranial nerve abnormalities, seizures and pseudocyst formation. More than half resolve completely although this may take up to 3 years. Most gamma knife centres (and more importantly their patients) accept an approximately 4% permanent complication rate.

Prediction of complications has been attempted using different models. The site of the nidus is an obvious factor [5]. Various mathematical models have attempted to refine this by factoring in the size of the AVM and the peripheral dose [3, 7, 12]. As might be expected, complication rates increase with larger radiation doses and treated volumes. The former can be adjusted in order to minimize the risk of radiation-induced side effects but only at the expense of lowering the success rate. Failure to obliterate the lesion would of course perpetuate the risk of haemorrhage, which carries its own morbidity – hence the need for a compromise in each case.

Two particular complications need separate mention. The concern is often raised whether ionising radiation may lead to delayed malignancy. So far the evidence suggests that this is extremely rare [10], to such an extent that an increased risk compared to the general population has not been demonstrated [8].

Pseudocyst formation several years after treatment has been described [9, 30]. Data from our own large database showed that the incidence is approximately 0.1% and in each case the normal brain around the target received an unusually high dose – caused by a difficulty with imaging, planning, targeting or that the treatment was a repeated irradiation for a large malformation. This observation suggests that the complication may well be avoidable.

The preparation for this review underlined the difficulties obtaining reliable data for publication. Even prospectively held large databases require retrospective maintenance. The difficulties finding the necessary data include lost follow up as a result of overseas residence, lack of interest by the patients and their physicians to adhere to protocols, refusing to undergo the gold standard angiography and patients moving away without forwarding address. There is also a tendency for successfully treated patients to become difficult to contact after the "closure" of a negative test whereas those requiring further treatment would return. Of course one can argue that some fatal bleeds may not be reported but accepted as sudden death by their carers. In spite of these uncertainties, one could demonstrate the usefulness of the method in a large number of cases.

Conclusions

Gamma knife radiosurgery for cerebral arteriovenous malformations has become an integral part of everyday neurosurgical practice. Departments offering a service for patients harbouring cerebral AVMs should have this modality available either locally or by a referral to a specialist centre. The latter may be facilitated by a networked solution or telemedicine. It is mandatory that before any treatment (other than emergency surgery for a haematoma) is undertaken, all modalities should be considered in a multidisciplinary fashion. A team with special interest and expertise in managing such cases should make the decisions, carry out the treatment(s) and follow up the patients. This arrangement will not only ensure a safe and efficient treatment but also allow feedback to monitor clinical results.

References

1. Chang SD, Marcellus ML, Marks MP, Levy RP, Do HM, Steinberg GK (2003) Multimodality treatment of giant intracranial arteriovenous malformations. Neurosurgery 53(1): 1–11
2. Coley SC, Wild JM, Wilkinson ID, Griffiths PD (2003) Neurovascular MRI with dynamic contrast-enhanced subtraction angiography. Neuroradiology 45(12): 843–850
3. Flickinger JC, Lunsford LD, Kondziolka D (1991) Dose-volume considerations in radiosurgery. Stereotact Funct Neurosurg 57(1–2): 99–105
4. Flickinger JC, Kondziolka D, Pollock BE, Maitz A, Lunsford LD (1997) Complications from arteriovenous malformation radiosurgery: Multivariate analysis and risk modeling. Int J Radiat Oncol Biol Phys 38: 485–490
5. Flickinger JC, Kondziolka D, Maitz AH, Lunsford LD (1998) Analysis of neurological sequelae from radiosurgery of arteriovenous malformations: how location affects outcome. Int J Radiat Oncol Biol Phys 15;40(2): 273–278
6. Flickinger JC, Kondziolka D, Lunsford LD *et al* (1999) A multi-institutional analysis of complication outcomes after arteriovenous malformation radiosurgery. Int J Radiat Oncol Biol Phys 44: 67–74
7. Flickinger JC, Kondziolka D, Lunsford LD, Kassam A, Phuong LK, Liscak R, Pollock B (2000) Development of a model to predict permanent symptomatic postradiosurgery injury for arteriovenous malformation patients. Arteriovenous Malformation Radiosurgery Study Group. Int J Radiat Oncol Biol Phys 15;46(5): 1143–1148
8. Ganz JC (2000) Gamma knife radiosurgery and its possible relationship to malignancy: a review. J Neurosurg 97 [Suppl] 5: 644–652
9. Hara M, Nakamura M, Shiokawa Y, Sawa H, Sato E, Koyasu H, Saito I (1998) Delayed cyst formation after radiosurgery for cerebral arteriovenous malformation: two case reports. Minim Invasive Neurosurg 41(1): 40–45
10. Kaido T, Hoshida T, Uranishi R, Akita N, Kotani A, Nishi N, Sakaki T (2001) Radiosurgery-induced brain tumor. Case report. J Neurosurg 95(4): 710–713
11. Karlsson B, Lindquist C, Steiner L (1996) Effect of gamma knife surgery on the risk of rupture prior to AVM obliteration. Minimally Invasive Neurosurgery 39(1): 21–27
12. Karlsson B, Lax I, Soderman M (1997) Factors influencing the risk for complications following gamma knife radiosurgery of cerebral arteriovenous malformations. Radiother Oncol 43(3): 275–280
13. Lai EH, Lun SL (2002) Impact on the quality of life of patients with arteriovenous malformations during the latent interval between gamma knife radiosurgery and lesion obliteration. J Neurosurg 97 [Suppl] 5: 471–473
14. Langer DJ, Lasner TM, Hurst RW, Flamm ES, Zager EL, King JT Jr (1998) Hypertension, small size, and deep venous drainage are associated with risk of hemorrhagic presentation of cerebral arteriovenous malformations. Neurosurgery 42(3): 481–486
15. Lawton MT, Hamilton MG, Spetzler RE (1995) Multimodality treatment of deep arteriovenous malformations: Thalamus, basal ganglia, and brain stem. Neurosurgery 37: 29–36
16. Major O, Szeifert GT, Fazekas I, Vitanovics D, Csonka E, Kocsis B, Bori Z, Kemeny AA, Nagy Z (2002) Effect of a single high-dose gamma irradiation on cultured cells in human cerebral arteriovenous malformation. J Neurosurg 97 [Suppl] 5: 459–463
17. Mori H, Aoki S, Okubo T, Hayashi N, Masumoto T, Yoshikawa T, Tago M, Shin M, Kurita H, Abe O, Ohtomo K (2003) Two-dimensional thick-slice MR digital subtraction angiography in the assessment of small to medium-size intracranial arteriovenous malformations. Neuroradiology 45(1): 27–33
18. Morgan MK, Drummond KJ, Grinnel IV, Sorby W (1997) Surgery for cerebral arteriovenous malformation: risks related to lenticulostriate arterial supply. J Neurosurg 86: 801–805
19. Pendl G, Unger F, Papaefthymiou G, Eustacchio S (2000) Staged radiosurgical treatment for large benign cerebral lesions. J Neurosurg 93 [Suppl] 3: 107–112
20. Pollock BE, Flickinger JC, Lunsford LD, Maitz A, Kondziolka D (1998) Factors associated with successful arteriovenous malformation radiosurgery. Neurosurgery 42(6): 1239–1244
21. Pollock BE (1998) Patient outcomes after arteriovenous malformation radiosurgery. In: Lunsford LD, Kondziolka D, Flickinger JC (eds) Gamma knife brain surgery. Prog Neurol Surg. Basel, Karger, vol 14, pp 51–59
22. Pollock BE, Kline RW, Stafford SL, Foote RL, Schomberg PJ (2000) The rationale and technique of staged-volume arteriovenous malformation radiosurgery. Int J Radiat Oncol Biol Phys 48(3): 817–824
23. Schneider BF, Eberhard DA, Steiner LE (1997) Histopathology of arteriovenous malformations after gamma knife radiosurgery. J Neurosurg 87(3): 352–357
24. Smith KA, Shetter A, Speiser B, Spetzler RF (1997) Angiographic follow-up in 37 patients after radiosurgery for cerebral arteriovenous malformations as part of a multimodality treatment approach. Stereotact Funct Neurosurg 69(1–4 Pt 2): 136–142
25. Steiner L, Leksell L, Greitz T, Forster DM, Backlund EO (1972) Stereotaxic radiosurgery for cerebral arteriovenous malformations. Report of a case. Acta Chir Scand 138(5): 459–464
26. Steiner L, Leksell L, Forster DM, Greitz T, Backlund EO (1974) Stereotactic radiosurgery in intracranial arterio-venous malformations. Acta Neurochirurgica (Wien) [Suppl] 21: 195–200
27. Szeifert G, Kemeny AA, Timperley WR, Forster DMC (1997) The potential role of myofibroblasts in arteriovenous malformation obliteration after radiosurgery. Neurosurgery 39(1): 67–70
28. Szeifert G, Kemeny AA, Major O, Timperley WR, Forster DMC (1998) Histopathological changes in cerebral arterio-

venous malformations following stereotactic irradiation with the gamma knife. In: Kondziolka D (ed) Radiosurgery 1997. Basel, Karger, vol 2, pp 129–136
29. Schaller C, Schramm J (1997) Microsurgical results for small arteriovenous malformations accessible for radiosurgical or embolization treatment. Neurosurgery 40(4): 664–672
30. Yamamoto M, Hara M, Ide M, Ono Y, Jimbo M, Saito I (1998) Radiation-related adverse effects observed on neuro-imaging several years after radiosurgery for cerebral arteriovenous malformations. Surg Neurol 49(4): 385–397

Correspondence: Andras A. Kemeny, FRCS M.D., National Centre for Stereotactic Radiosurgery, Royal Hallamshire Hospital, Glossop Road, S10 2JF Sheffield, U.K. e-mail: a.kemeny@shef.ac.uk

Acta Neurochir (2004) [Suppl] 91: 65–74

Gamma knife radiosurgery of skull base meningiomas

R. Liščák[1,2], A. Kollová[1], V. Vladyka[1], G. Šimonová[1], and J. Novotný Jr[1]

[1] Department of Stereotactic and Radiation Neurosurgery, Na Homolce Hospital, Prague, Czech Republic
[2] Department of Neurosurgery, III. Faculty of Medicine, Charles University, Prague, Czech Republic

Summary

Meningiomas are the most frequent benign tumors treated by gamma knife radiosurgery and the majority of them are located on the skull base. Between 1992 and 1999, 197 skull base-located meningiomas in 192 patients were treated by gamma knife in Prague. Contact with the chiasma or optic tract was not regarded as a contraindication for gamma knife radiosurgery and such contact was observed in 32% of the skull base meningiomas treated. 176 patients were monitored during a median of 36 months, of whom 73% showed a decrease in tumor volume; no change was observed in 25% and continued growth was observed in 2%. Neurodeficit improved in 63% of patients, temporary morbidity occurred in 11% and persistent morbidity remained in 4.5%. Radiosurgery induced edema in 11%. Significantly lower edema occurrence was observed after radiosurgery in patients with no history of edema prior to radiosurgery, where the tumor was located in the posterior skull base and where the dosage to the tumor margin was lower than or equal to 14 Gy. Radiosurgery of skull base meningiomas has been proven to be safe and efficient. We consider gamma knife treatment for skull base meningiomas to be the method of choice whenever tumors are within the volume limits and there is no need for an urgent decompressive effect from the open operation.

Keywords: Meningiomas; skull base; gamma knife; radiosurgery.

Introduction

Meningiomas represent about 17–30% of all intracranial neoplasms and their incidence in the population is reported to be between 1 and 6 per 100,000 people [8]. The incidence of meningiomas increases with age and radiosurgery is a welcome treatment option for internally debilitated patients. Meningiomas are currently the most frequently treated benign tumors using gamma knife radiosurgery. Previously, close contact with the optic tract was considered to be a contraindication for radiosurgery of skull base meningiomas [9, 14, 53], however this limitation should no longer be considered absolute. Positive results have been obtained using gamma knife treatment where tumor control was achieved with no attendant complications, even in cases of optic tract compression caused by meningioma [29]. Thus many patients, who were not previously considered candidates for radiosurgery, could profit from gamma knife treatment with no higher risk of morbidity than patients with tumors distant from the optic tract.

Materials and methods

Between 1992 and 2003, 873 patients with meningioma were treated in Prague's Na Homolce Hospital using the Leksell gamma knife. This represented 17.3% of all treated patients. Patients treated before 1999 were analyzed. Patients with malignant meningiomas (atypical or anaplastic) and patients with neurofibromatosis were excluded, leaving 389 meningiomas in 349 patients to be treated with the gamma knife. This group of patients included 197 meningiomas in 192 individuals located at the skull base, and these composed the target group for this paper. Thus, patients with skull base meningiomas represent 55% of all treated meningiomas. In this group of 192 patients there was a predominance of women to men, with a ratio of 4:1. The patients' age ranged from 23 to 82 years, median 60 years. Gamma knife radiosurgery was the primary treatment for 66% of patients. 34% of patients had previously undergone open surgery, and in 3% this was followed by fractionated radiotherapy. In 51% of treated cases the meningioma extended into the cavernous sinus, in 15% it was intrasellar, in 15% the sphenoid wing was involved, in 4% it had spread into the orbita, the anterior skull base was involved in 6%, in 21% it had spread to the clivus and the pontocerebellar angle was involved in 25%. Contact with the chiasm or optic tract was not considered a contraindication for gamma knife radiosurgery and this contact was observed in 32% of skull base meningiomas treated (Figs. 1, 2). Compression of the brain stem by meningioma was observed in 37% of cases (Fig. 2).

Radiosurgery under local anesthesia was performed using the Leksell gamma knife (Elekta Instrument AB). CT was used to localize the tumor in the first 27 patients, MRI was then used in all other patients. A T1-weighted, contrast-enhanced spin echo (SE) sequence in both axial and coronal planes, slice thickness 3 mm, was performed on Magnetom Impact Expert 1.0 Tesla (Siemens) equipment for target definition. All the sequences used for stereotactic localization were tested using phantom studies and the linearity of the

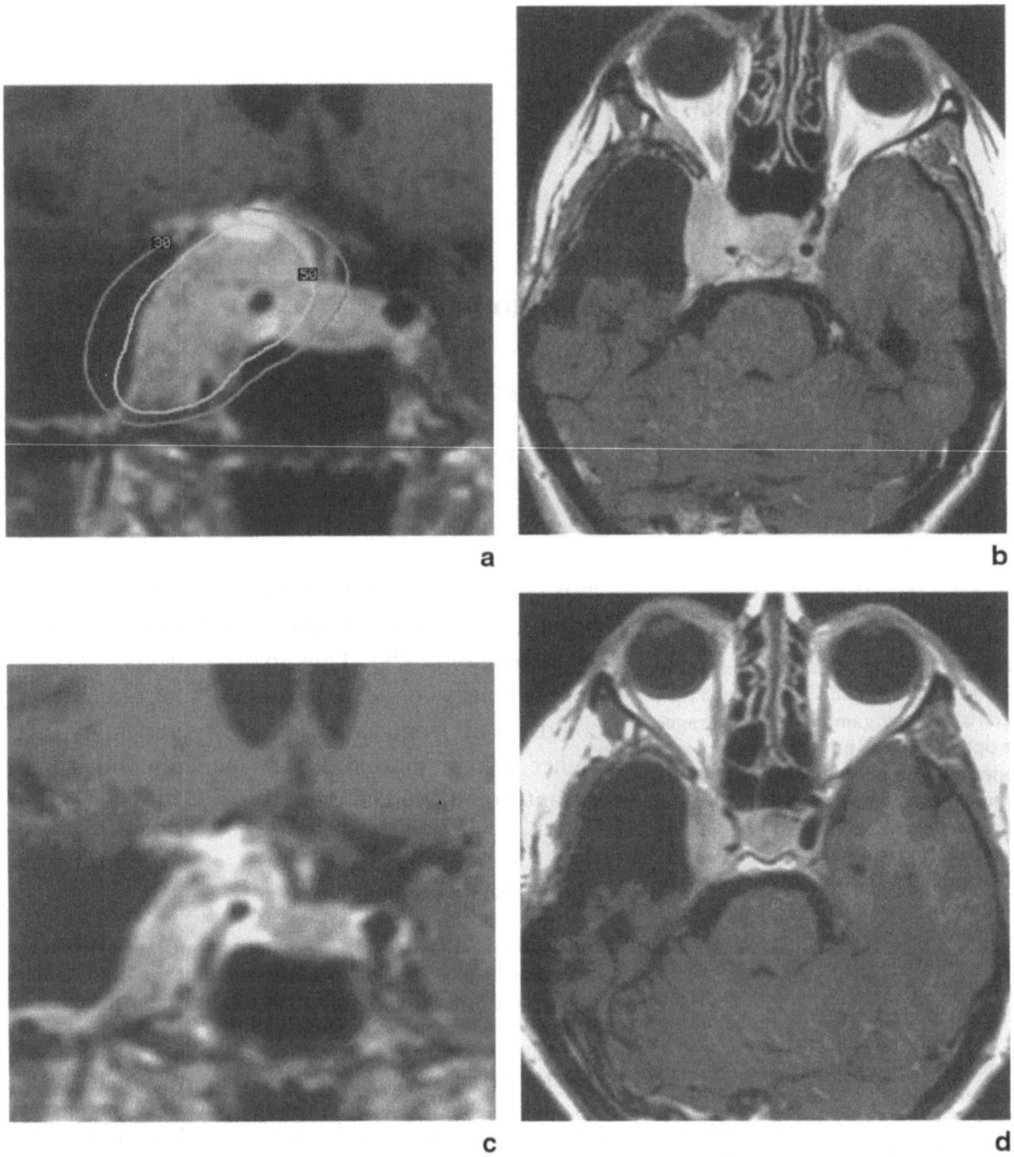

Fig. 1. (a,b) 47-year-old woman with tumor progression 3 years after a previous partial resection, gamma knife radiosurgery with a marginal dose of 12 Gy and a 50% isodose, maximum dose to the opticus 8 Gy. (c,d) 7 years after radiosurgery, decrease in tumor volume, no treatment-related morbidity

magnetic field was guaranteed [36]. The KULA planning system (Elekta Instrument AB) was used to plan the radiation dose delivery for the first 12 patients, while the Gamma Plan (Elekta Instrument AB) planning system was used for the remainder.

The volume of the skull base meningiomas ranged between 0.12 and 36.5 cm^3, median 5.3 cm^3. The minimal marginal dose ranged from 6.5 to 20.4 Gy, median 12 Gy. This dose was delivered in a 40–80%, median 50% isodose. Thus the maximum dose was between 13 and 36 Gy, median 24 Gy. Because of the size of the meningioma volume in 9 patients, radiosurgery was performed in two stages at least 6 months apart. For the single stage procedure, the number of isocenters ranged from 1–17, median 8. Where vision had been preserved, the dose to the optic tract did not exceed 8 Gy and the dose to the brain stem was below 14 Gy. Where the tumor was in contact with the optic nerve but vision had been preserved, the small rim of the meningioma adjacent to the optic tract was covered with a lower isodose, while the rest of the tumor was covered with a 50% isodose. No higher than a 35% isodose was used to irradiate the optic tract and the optic apparatus was not exposed to a dose of more than 8 Gy (Figs. 1, 2). This dose was only exceeded in cases where blindness had previously occurred as a result of the disease or previous surgery (Fig. 3). In the cases of patients who had previously undergone fractionated radiotherapy, the dose to the optic apparatus did not exceed 3 Gy. Where necessary, some source segments were plugged in order to stay within this tolerance limit. Other surrounding structures are more radiation-resistant in comparison to the optic nerve and their relation to the meningioma is not generally regarded as a limit to radiosurgery.

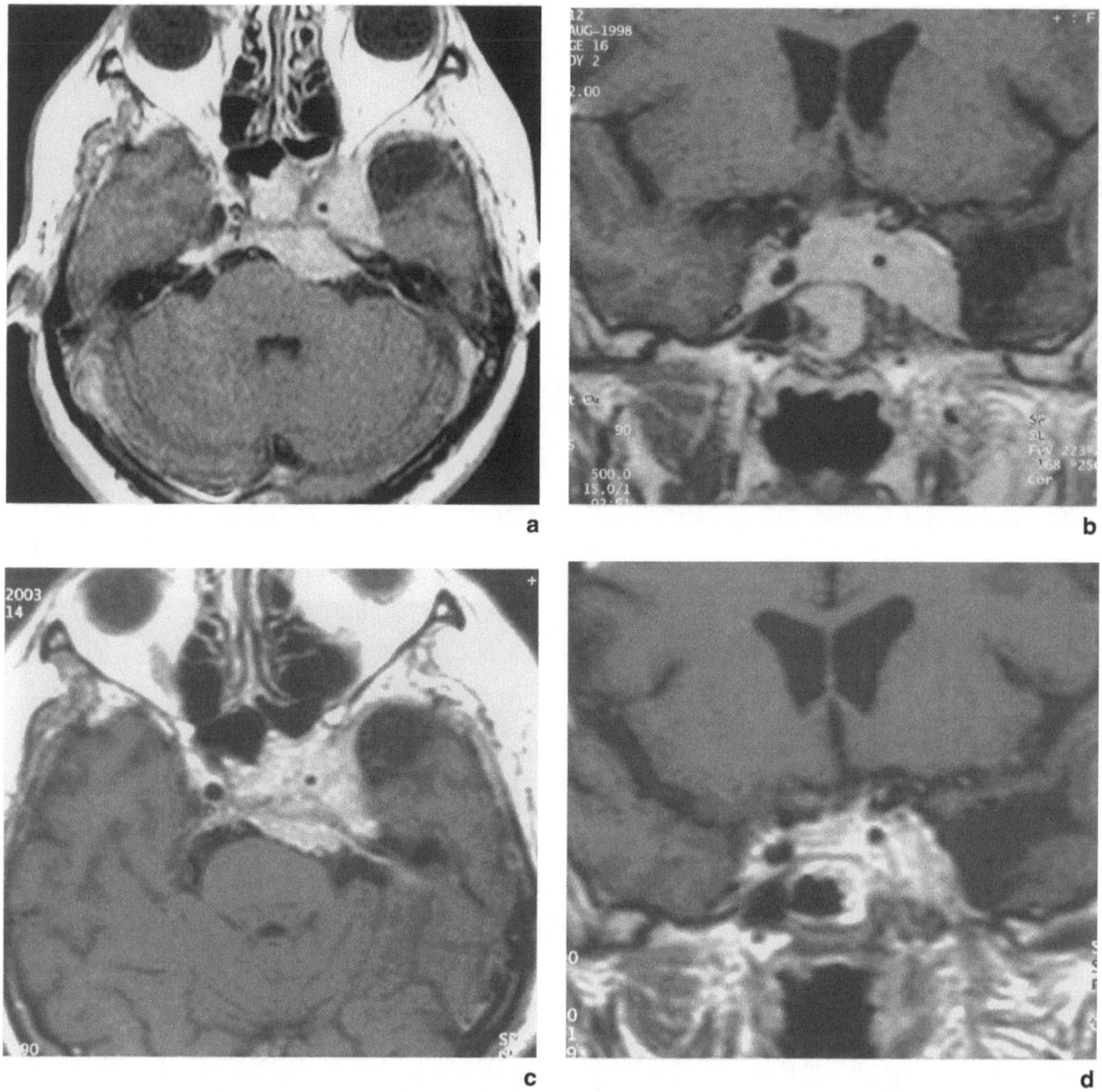

Fig. 2. (a,b) 61-year-old female, after 3 open surgeries (2 surgeries reported as radical resections and one as a removal of a postoperative epidural hematoma), tumor progression with the ophtalmoplegia on the left side, gamma knife radiosurgery performed with a marginal dose of 12 Gy and a 50% isodose. (c,d) 5 years after radiosurgery, decrease in tumor volume, no treatment-related morbidity

Results

Of a group of 192 patients, we lost contact with 7 patients (they either moved without providing a new address or refused follow-up) and 15 patients died (4 of cancer, 3 of heart failure, 2 of ictus and 6 for unknown reasons). The remaining 176 patients were monitored for a median of 36 months, ranging from 6 to 110 months.

Tumor volume decrease was detected in 129 (73%) patients 6–110 months after gamma knife treatment, median 24 months (Figs. 1–3). No change in tumor volume was observed in 44 (25%) patients. Continued tumor growth was observed in 3 (2%) of patients 12–38 months after treatment. Gamma knife treatment was repeated in one of these patients, fractionated radiotherapy was recommended for another and the third underwent subsequent open surgery with frac-

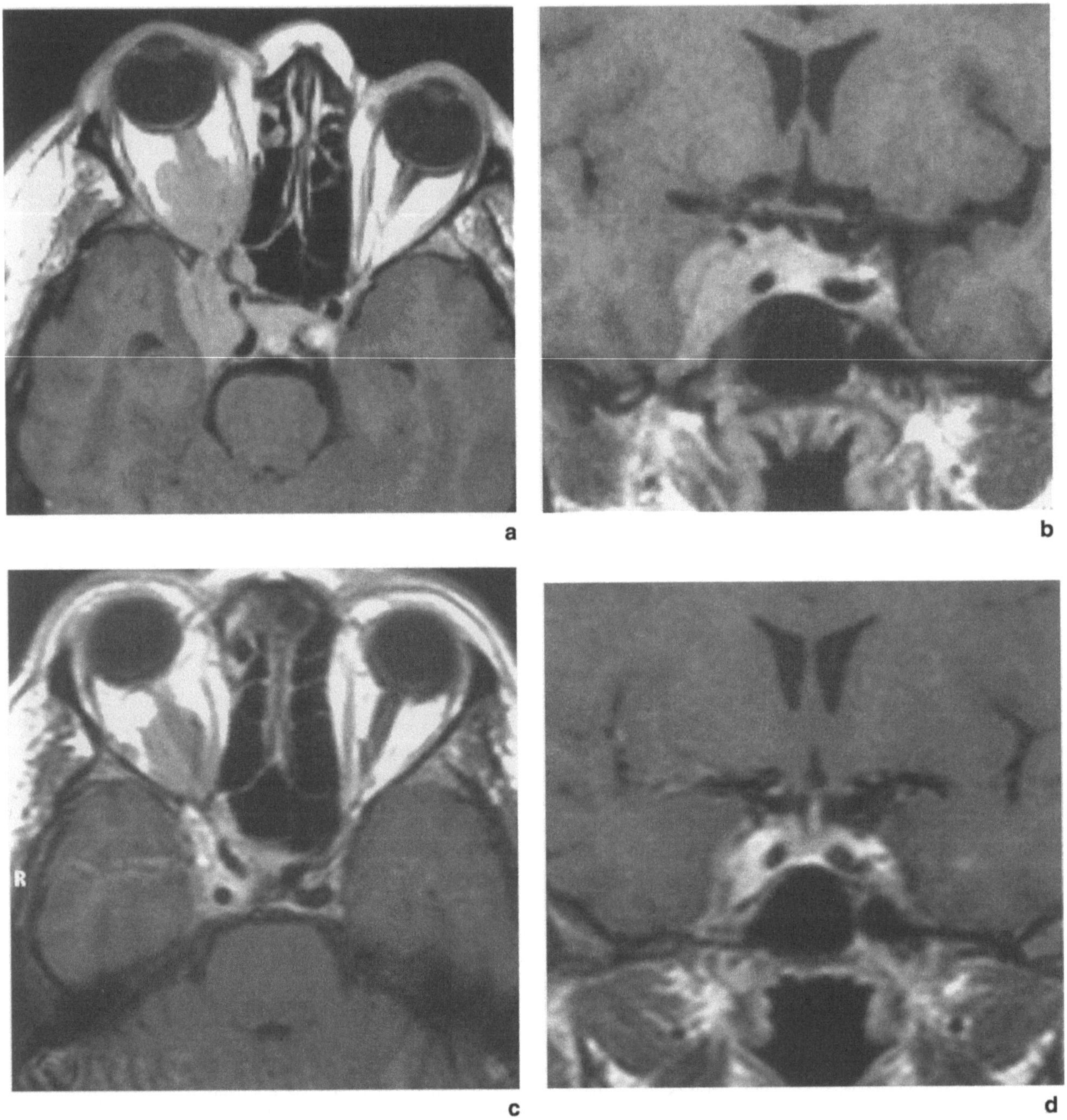

Fig. 3. (a,b) 47-year-old female, after 2 open surgeries, tumor progression with ophtalmoplegia and blindness on the right side, gamma knife radiosurgery performed with a marginal dose of 12 Gy and a 50% isodose. (c,d) 8 years after radiosurgery, decrease in tumor volume

tionated radiotherapy. Neurodeficit, which was present prior to the gamma knife radiosurgery, improved in 111 patients (63%). Headaches were relieved in 71 patients, oculomotor nerve palsy in 31 patients, neuropathy of the trigeminal nerve in 31 patients, facial nerve palsy in 10 patients, hearing improved in 6 patients, psychosyndrome in 3 patients, lack of balance in 21 patients, hemiparesis in 11 patients and visual function in 24 patients. In the case of primary radiosurgery, this improvement was connected with tumor volume decrease. In cases where open surgery had previously taken place, the ongoing rehabilitation of the postoperative deficit could also play a contributing role. The neurodeficit was impaired after gamma knife radiosurgery in 19 patients (11%) from 0.5 to 48, median 5 months after the treatment. Among these patients impairment of psychosyndrome was observed in 2, oculomotor nerve deficit in 5, neuropathy of the trigeminal nerve in 9, impairment of vertigo in 2 and impaired epilepsy in 1 patient. In 12 of these patients collateral edema induced by radiosurgery was detected. This morbidity had a tendency to improve and so far has resolved in 11 patients between 12 and 98, median 24 months after treatment. Persistent morbidity remained in 8 patients (4.5%).

12 (6%) patients were suffering from epilepsy before radiosurgery and in 8 of these the epilepsy improved after treatment. Another 3 patients had experienced some isolated seizures before radiosurgery, which were not repeated after gamma knife radiosurgery. In 1 patient, epilepsy that worsened 3 months after radiosurgery due to the induced collateral edema, later resolved and by the last follow-up, 54 months after radiosurgery, there was an overall improvement in epileptic seizures.

Collateral edema before treatment was detected in 5 patients (3%). Radiosurgery induced edema in 19 patients (11%), which was detected 1–36, median 12 months after radiosurgery. In 7 of these patients edema was asymptomatic, whereas symptoms caused by edema were present in 12 patients (7%). These symptomatic cases of edema were observed earlier, 1–12, median 5 months after radiosurgery and symptoms have so far been resolved in 8 patients by 2–44, median 12 months after radiosurgery. Induced collateral edema had a tendency to resolve and to date has completely resolved in 10 patients by 7–44, median 18 months after radiosurgery. At the time the gamma knife radiosurgery was undertaken, 11 patients were under corticoid medication, usually initiated after their previous open surgery and 7 of these were able to abandon this medication after the gamma knife radiosurgery. In the 12 patients with symptomatic edema after radiosurgery, corticoids were administered for periods ranging between 0.5 and 18, median 4 months.

Statistical analysis

To discover how various factors influenced the radiosurgical treatment of skull base meningiomas using the gamma knife, a total of ten different variables were proposed. These factors included pretreatment variables: the patient's sex and age, whether patient had previously undergone open surgery, whether neurodeficit and collateral edema were present before radiosurgery, whether the margin of the tumor was lobulated and tumor enhancement heterogeneous, and the tumor volume and location of meningioma (fossa cranii anterior, media and posterior). Treatment variables included: the maximal dose to the meningioma and the dose to the meningioma margin.

Altogether five different events after gamma knife radiosurgery were studied as potentially dependent on these proposed factors. The events were as follows: decrease or increase in tumor volume, occurrence of post-irradiation collateral edema, improvement or worsening of the neurodeficit after radiosurgery.

To point out those factors influencing the time dependence of the events listed above, univariate and multivariate statistical analysis methods were employed. Univariate analysis was performed using Kaplan-Meier statistics with a log rank test. Multivariate analysis was performed with the Cox proportional hazards model using the backward stepwise (conditional likelihood ratio) method. The analyses were performed using the SPSS statistical software version 10.0. Variables with significant p-values ($p < 0.05$) in at least one of two actuarial analyses were considered possible risk factors for the event.

The summary of the statistical analysis results is given in Table 1. Factors having a significant influence on the studied events are indicated and the significant p-values are listed for both the univariate and multivariate analyses.

A significantly higher incidence of tumor volume decrease was observed in patients who had not undergone previous surgery ($p = 0.028$ Log Rank). The cumulative tumor control rate (no change or decrease of tumor volume) after radiosurgery is given in Graph 1.

Significantly lower edema occurrence after radiosurgery was observed in patients who had previously undergone surgery ($p = 0.030$ Log Rank), as well as for patients who had no history of edema prior to radiosurgery ($p < 0.001$ Log Rank, $p = 0.006$ Cox), where the tumor was located in the posterior skull base ($p = 0.029$ Log Rank, $p = 0.041$ Cox) and where doses to the tumor margin were lower or equal to 14 Gy ($p = 0.035$ Log Rank, $p = 0.005$ Cox) – Graphs 2, 3.

No significant influence of any proposed factors was observed on tumor volume increase or the improvement or worsening of the neurodeficit after radiosurgery.

Table 1. *Summary of statistical analysis results. Factors having a significant influence on the studied events are indicated and significant p-values are listed for both univariate and multivariate analysis. Univariate analysis was performed using Kaplan-Meier statistics with a log rank test. Multivariate analysis was performed with the Cox proportional hazards model using the backward stepwise (conditional likelihood ratio) method*

Factors	Tumor decrease	Tumor increase	Edema occurrence	Neurodeficit improvement	Neurodeficit impairment
Sex	x	x	x	x	x
Age	x	x	x	x	x
Previous surgery	p = 0.028 (Log Rank)	x	p = 0.030 (Log Rank)	x	x
Edema before LGKS	x	x	p < 0.001 (Log Rank) p = 0.006 (Cox)	x	x
Lobulated margin	x	x	x	x	x
Heterogeneity	x	x	x	x	x
Tumor volume	x	x	x	x	x
Tumor location	x	x	p = 0.029 (Log Rank) p = 0.041 (Cox)	x	x
Dose to max	x	x	x	x	x
Dose to margin	x	x	p = 0.035 (Log Rank) p = 0.005 (Cox)	x	x

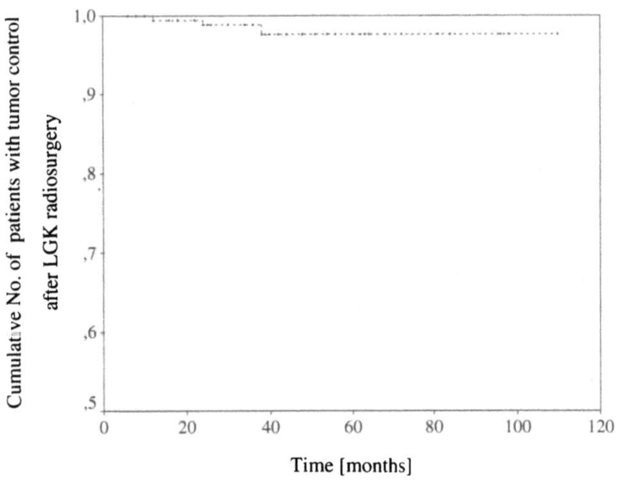

Graph 1. Kaplan-Meier curve for the cumulative tumor control rate (no change or decrease in the tumor volume) after LGK radiosurgery

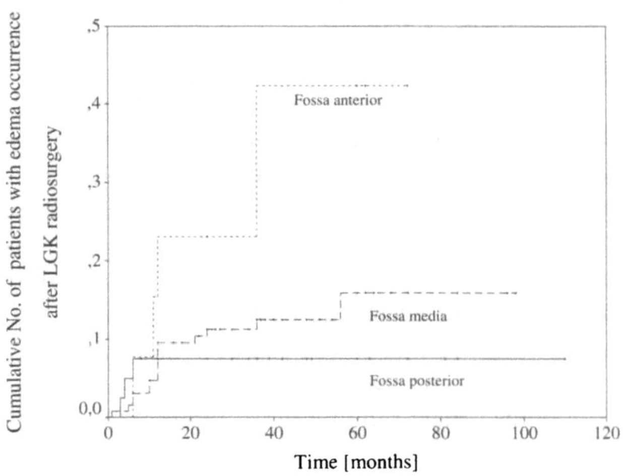

Graph 2. Kaplan-Meier curves for the cumulative number of patients with edema occurrence after LGK radiosurgery for different meningioma locations

Discussion

Radiosurgery was first introduced by the Swedish neurosurgeon Lars Leksell in 1951 [26]. Because of its historical background, radiosurgery has been incorporated into the field of neurosurgery and it shares common features with neurosurgical operations. Firstly, radiosurgery uses principles of stereotactic neurosurgery with the same co-ordinate frame attached to the patient's head and the same principles of targeting the pathological lesion as in any other stereotactic neurosurgical procedure. Secondly, focused radiation with a selective effect on the target relies on detailed neuroanatomical knowledge, which forms part of neurosurgical training. Thirdly, radiosurgery, just like any other operation, is a single session procedure. However, fundamental differences exist between it and an open neurosurgical operation. Firstly, radiosurgery is a non-invasive procedure, which avoids all the risks associated with open procedures (bleeding, infection, cerebrospinal fluid fistula, etc.). Secondly, except in the case of small children, radiosurgery is performed under local anesthesia, thus avoiding all the risks inherent in general anesthetics (particularly important for internally debilitated patients). Thirdly, open operation and radiosurgery achieve the same

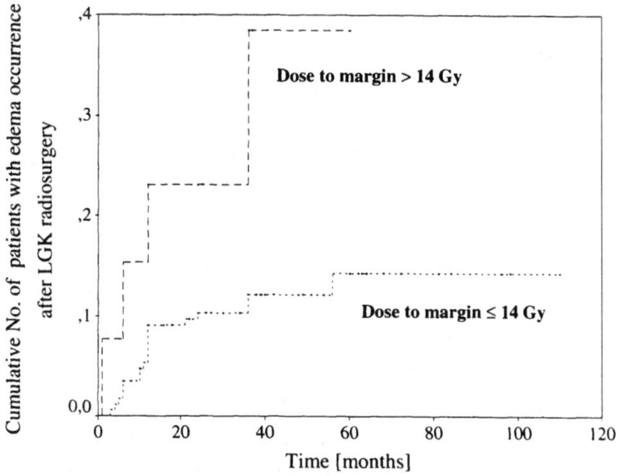

Graph 3. Kaplan-Meier curves for the cumulative number of patients with edema occurrence after LGK radiosurgery for different marginal doses to the meningioma

goal in fundamentally different ways. The common goal is to spare the patient's life, which is threatened by a growing tumor. While open operation achieves this goal through radical resection and anatomical removal of the tumor, radiosurgery leaves the tumor in place. Radiosurgery achieves sterilization of the tumor and this method is successful if the tumor cells lose their potential to make colonies of daughter cells. During the follow-up the tumor may still be visible, but does not continue to grow and ceases to represent a threat to the patient. In some patients regression and decrease of tumor size after radiosurgery can be detected, which is a bonus for the patient. However, this decompressive effect cannot be guaranteed in advance in radiosurgery.

Its use of radiation makes radiosurgery interdisciplinary with radiotherapy and a radiation oncologist is a member of the radiosurgical team. Similarly to neurosurgery, radiosurgery has some features in common with, and others different from, radiotherapy. Radiosurgery shares with radiotherapy the use of radiation to cure the patient, which demands the same general radiohygienic arrangements. Radiosurgery using the gamma knife requires the same safety precautions as any other radiotherapeutic procedure. However, there are significant differences between radiosurgery and radiotherapy and these derive from the fact that radiosurgery is a single session delivery of focused radiation, while radiotherapy is prescribed in many fractions. Radiosurgery delivers a high focused radiation dose to the tumor with a steep fall-off of the dose, thus sparing the surrounding normal brain tissue. Radiotherapy presents a less conformal irradiation and a significant volume of normal surrounding brain tissue receives the same radiation dose as the tumor during fractionated radiotherapy. A radiation dose applied in a single fraction creates a significantly higher radiobiological effect as compared to the same dose delivered in many fractions [19]. One of the reasons for fractionation in radiotherapy is the lower conformity of the irradiation, because fractionation spares more late responding tissue (brain), than earlier responding tissue (tumor). The radiosensitivity of the tumor tissue provides a therapeutic window for fractionated radiotherapy. Radioresistant tumors (typically benign tumors) have a lower alpha/beta ratio (from a linear quadratic model of cell survival), which is advantageous to use single fraction radiosurgery [24]. Radiosurgery, therefore, overrides the limits of radiosensitivity and, in the case of benign tumors, the control rate after radiosurgery is comparable to a radical resection of the tumor; while fractionated radiotherapy is a more or less palliative treatment [27]. Compared to fractionated radiotherapy, radiosurgery is limited by the volume of the tumor. In the case of the radiobiologically powerful single session irradiation, the risk of radionecrosis is volume dependent [10]. In some cases, the close connection of the tumor to specific functionally important structures can represent another limit to radiosurgery. Considering the marginal dose used for meningiomas, which is usually at least 12 Gy and the tolerance of functionally important structures, the most decisive limit is the relation of the tumor to the optic tract [25, 53]. At the beginning of our clinical experience with radiosurgery we rejected patients with meningiomas touching the optic tract, unless the affected side was blind. When prescribing radiosurgery for patients suffering from blindness we frequently observed that this was a complication resulting from previous surgery, when radiosurgery had not been considered as a primary treatment because vision was preserved at the time the meningioma was diagnosed. We later changed this strategy in cases concerning elderly patients, where invasive treatment was not possible. Experience showing that when a small rim adjacent to the optic tract was covered with a lower dose, no visual impairment resulted and that the tumor control rate was preserved, and this method now allows us to offer radiosurgery as a choice to all patients with skull base meningiomas, regardless of their distance from the optic tract. The only cases where radiosurgery is not now indicated are cases of preserved vision, where there is orbital spread of the tumor and the optic nerve passing through the mass of the tumor.

The role of radiosurgery must be considered while taking into account fractionated radiotherapy and microsurgery. There is no consensus of opinion concerning fractionated radiotherapy of meningiomas. For the most part, fractionated radiotherapy is accepted as a treatment that prevents or postpones recurrence of subtotally extirpated meningiomas [13]. Radiotherapy is not recommended for radically removed meningiomas [12, 33]. The opinion that fractionated radiotherapy of meningiomas is of dubious value is less common, but serious complications were reported in 56 to 75% of all subtotally resected meningiomas, and radiated meningiomas recurred during follow up [32, 56]. In spite of the fact that fractionated radiotherapy is accepted as an adjuvant therapy for residual meningiomas [30], it is at the same time a significant risk factor for the appearance of radiation induced meningiomas [4, 16, 55]. To our knowledge, there has been no published evidence of a radiation induced meningioma occurring after radiosurgery. As for benign tumors, radiosurgery should be preferred over fractionated radiotherapy for radiobiological reasons. Benign tumors are relatively radioresistant and fractionated radiotherapy of small and circumscribed tumors is not justifiable if gamma knife radiosurgery or any type of stereotactic radiosurgery is available.

The process of deciding between radiosurgery and microsurgery must be stratified. Microsurgery of skull base meningiomas, despite improved techniques, still remains a risky procedure. Open resection of skull base meningiomas carries the risk of mortality and postoperative impairment of the quality of life and even the radical resection cannot prevent recurrence in all patients [6, 7, 31, 38, 46, 57]. Complete resection of skull base meningiomas is not always possible and in 16 papers encompassing a total of 1,028 patients, complete resection was reported in 17 to 96%, median of 62% of cases, morbidity was reported in 0 to 45%, median 20% and mortality was 0 to 16%, median 3.5% [2, 3, 5–7, 17, 20, 21, 31, 38, 42–45, 59, 60]. Nevertheless, the quality of life after surgery could be worse then reported and the burden on the patient's caregiver is profound, with 43–75% of surviving patients who underwent surgery for petroclival meningiomas functioning below accepted norms and 56% of caregivers (usually close relatives) experiencing major changes in their lifestyle [23]. The patients' quality of life should be preserved at all costs, and when this aim cannot be fulfilled by microsurgery, radiosurgery can be carried out as a primary modality or in addition to microsurgery [49].

Radiosurgery of skull base meningiomas has been proven to be safe and efficient. In 10 papers reporting gamma knife treatment of skull base meningiomas and covering 556 patients, treatment mortality was zero and morbidity ranged from 0 to 8%, median 4% and tumor control was achieved in 90–100%, median 96% [1, 9, 18, 22, 34, 40, 41, 47, 50, 52]. Meningiomas in this location do not have a tendency to induce huge or intractable collateral edema, especially when the marginal dose is kept below 15 Gy, which is also recommended for meningiomas on the skull convexity [28]. The lower incidence of collateral edema observed in the posterior skull base is in accordance with general experience. Therefore we see a therapeutic window for a marginal dose to benign meningiomas of between 12 and 15 Gy. This dose range kept the tumor control rate above 97%. The marginal dose below 12 Gy was only applied in cases of previous fractionated radiotherapy in our series.

We consider gamma knife treatment for skull base meningiomas to be the method of choice whenever the tumors fall within the volume limits. A different situation occurs with meningiomas located on the skull convexity, which deserve a more cautious approach when prescribing gamma knife radiosurgery. Meningiomas are typically highly vascular tumors and one of the factors involved in vasculogenesis – vascular endothelial growth factor (VEGF) is also a potent inducer of vascular permeability and seems to be a primary mediator of peritumoral edema [15]. Release of this factor from tumor cells damaged by the radiation could induce more significant edema, when there is no thin layer of space filled with liquor and VEGF can directly influence the adjacent brain tissue. Tumor infiltration into the adjacent brain tissue and pial-cortical blood supply are critical factors for the development of peritumoral brain edema among patients with meningiomas [51]. Convexity meningiomas are mostly not cleavable tumors, intimately touching the brain surface [48], while the surface of skull base meningiomas is more significantly in contact with cistern space as compared to convexity meningiomas. Therefore convexity meningiomas could have a higher propensity to induce more significant collateral edema, which can sometimes be observed, especially when a higher marginal dose is applied [11, 28, 39]. In this location radiosurgery is recommended, if microsurgery is contraindicated for any reason or the tumor infiltrates sinuses and their radical resection is not possible.

The question remains as to whether any type of treatment, including radiosurgery, should be prescribed for incidentally diagnosed meningiomas. Meningioma is a slow-growing tumor and to prove its growth, it is often necessary to observe the patient for more than 10 years [31]. Olivero *et al.* [37] presented a group of 45 patients with asymptomatic meningiomas. They observed no growth in 35 patients during a follow up period lasting an average of 29 months, while in 10 patients (22%) over an average follow up period of 47 months, they monitored average growths of 2.4 mm annually, up to a maximum of 10 mm annually. Van Havenbergh *et al.* [54] monitored 21 patients with petroclival meningioma for at least 4 years, and observed growth in 76% and functional deterioration in 63%. While a "wait and see policy" can exclude some patients from risky open surgery, when applied to radiosurgery, this strategy gradually disqualifies all patients for this kind of non-invasive treatment, or at the very least make it more complicated. Therefore this option can only be recommended in cases where regular follow up is available. Access to repeated MRI is not easy to organize for all referring physicians. Therefore we advocate a conservative approach to incidentally diagnosed convexity meningiomas for older patients (depending on their biological status) or patients with calcified tumors and atrophic brains. These patients could be followed and active treatment could be indicated only when progression and growth of the tumor is observed [35, 58]. In the case of skull base meningiomas it is better to indicate low risk non-invasive radiosurgery when the meningioma is small and distant from the optic tract than to wait until the tumor grows too large for radiosurgery and open surgery is too risky for the patient.

Gamma knife radiosurgery of meningiomas is playing an increasingly important role in Czech neurosurgery. In 2001, 417 patients with meningiomas were treated by open resection in all 18 neurosurgical departments in the Czech Republic, while 97 patients were treated by gamma knife during the same year, representing 19% of all patients with meningiomas treated neurosurgically. In 2002, 130 patients with meningiomas were treated using the gamma knife and 448 patients were treated by open surgery, thus gamma knife radiosurgery represented 22.5% of all neurosurgically treated patients in the Czech Republic with this diagnosis.

References

1. Aichholzer M, Bertalanffy A, Dietrich W *et al* (2000) Gamma knife radiosurgery of skull base meningiomas. Acta Neurochir (Wien) 142: 647–653
2. Al-Mefty O (1990) Clinoidal meningiomas. J Neurosurg 73: 840–849
3. Arai H, Sato K, Okuda *et al* (2000) Transcranial transsphenoidal approach for tuberculum sellae meningiomas. Acta Neurochir (Wien) 142: 751–757
4. Brada M, Ford D, Ashley S *et al* (1992) Risk of second brain tumor after conservative surgery and radiotherapy for pituitary adenoma. BMJ 304(6838): 1343–1346
5. Ciric I, Landau B (1993) Tentorial and posterior cranial fossa meningiomas: operative results and long-term follow-up: experience with twenty-six cases. Surg Neurol 39(6): 530–537
6. De Jesús O, Sekhar LN, Parikh HK, Wright DC, Wagner DP (1996) Long-term follow up of patients with meningiomas involving the cavernous sinus: recurrence, progression, and quality of life. Neurosurgery 39: 915–920
7. DeMonte F, Smith HK, Al-Mefty O (1994) Outcome of aggressive removal of cavernous sinus meningiomas. J Neurosurg 81(2): 245–251
8. DeMonte F, Marmor E, Al-Mefty O (2001) Meningiomas. In: Kaye AH, Laws ER Jr (eds) Brain tumors. Churchill Livingstone, London, pp 719–750
9. Duma CM, Lunsford LD, Kondziolka D, Harsh IV GR, Flickinger JC (1993) Stereotactic radiosurgery of cavernous sinus meningiomas as an addition or alternative to microsurgery. Neurosurgery 32(5): 699–705
10. Flickinger JC, Lunsford LD, Kondziolka D (1992) Dose prescription and dose volume effects in radiosurgery. Neurosurg Clin North Am 3(1): 51–59
11. Ganz JC, Schrottner O, Pendl G (1996) Radiation-induced edema after gamma knife treatment for meningioma. Stereotact Funct Neurosurg 66 [Suppl] 1: 129–133
12. Glaholm J, Bloom HJ, Crow JH (1990) The role of radiotherapy in the management of intracranial meningiomas. Int J Radiat Oncol Biol Phys 18(4): 755–761
13. Goldsmith BJ, Wara WM, Wilson ChB, Larson DA (1994) Postoperative irradiation for subtotally resected meningiomas. J Neurosurg 80: 192–201
14. Hakim R, Alexander III E, Loeffler JS *et al* (1998) Results of linear accelerator-based radiosurgery for intracranial meningiomas. Neurosurgery 42: 446–454
15. Harrigan MR (2003) Angiogenic factors in the central nervous system. Neurosurgery 53: 639–661
16. Harrison MJ, Wolfe DE, Lau TS, Mitnick RJ, Sachdev VP (1991) Radiation induced meningiomas: experience at the Mount Sinai Hospital and review of the literature. J Neurosurg 75(4): 564–574
17. Honeybul S, Neil-Dwyer G, Lang DA, Evans BT, Ellison DW (2001) Sphenoid wing meningioma en plaque: a clinical review. Acta Neurochir (Wien) 143(8): 749–758
18. Iwai Y, Yamanaka K, Ishiguro T (2003) Gamma knife radiosurgery for the treatment of cavernous sinus meningiomas. Neurosurgery 52: 517–524
19. Joiner MC (1993) The linear-quadratic approach to fractionation. In: Steel GG (ed) Basic clinical radiobiology for radiation oncologist. Edward Arnold Publishers, London

20. Kim DK, Grieve J, Archer DJ, Uttley D (1996) Meningiomas in the region of the cavernous sinus: a review of 21 patients. Br J Neurosurg 10(5): 439–444
21. Kleinpeter G, Bock F (1990) Invasion of the cavernous sinus by medial sphenoid meningioma-"radical" surgery and recurrence. Acta Neurochir (Wien) 103(3–4): 87–91
22. Kurita H, Sasaki T, Kawamoto S *et al* (1997) Role of radiosurgery in the management of cavernous sinus meningiomas. Acta Neurol Scand 96(5): 297–304
23. Lang DA, Neil-Dwyer G, Garfield J (1999) Outcome after complex neurosurgery: the caregiver's burden is forgotten. J Neurosurg 91: 359–363
24. Larson DA, Flickinger JC, Loefler JS (1993) The radiobiology of radiosurgery. Int J Radiation Oncology Biol Phys 2: 557–561
25. Leber KA, Bergloff J, Pendl G (1998) Dose response tolerance of the visual pathways and cranial nerves of the cavernous sinus to stereotactic radiosurgery. J Neurosurg 88: 43–50
26. Leksell L (1951) The stereotactic method and radiosurgery of the brain. Acta Chir Scand 102: 316–319
27. Linskey ME (2000) Stereotactic radiosurgery versus stereotactic radiotherapy for patients with vestibular schwannoma: a Leksell gamma knife society 2000 debate. J Neurosurg [Suppl] 3(93): 90–95
28. Liscak R, Vladyka V, Simonova G, Novotny J Jr, Syrucek M (1998) Gamma-knife radiosurgery of meningiomas – preliminary results and complications. J Radiosurgery 1: 35–42
29. Liscak R, Simonova G, Vymazal J, Janouskova L, Vladyka V (1999) Gamma knife radiosurgery of meningiomas in the cavernous sinus region. Acta Neurochir (Wien) 141: 473–480
30. Lunsford LD (1994) Contemporary management of meningiomas: radiation therapy as an adjuvant and radiosurgery as an alternative to surgical removal? J Neurosurg 80: 187–190
31. Mathiesen T, Lindquist C, Kihlstrom L, Karlsson B (1996) Recurrence of cranial base meningiomas. Neurosurgery 39: 2–9
32. Mathiesen T, Kihlstrom, Karlsson B, Lindquist Ch (2003) Potential complications following radiotherapy for meningiomas. Surg Neurol 60: 193–200
33. Miralbell R, Linggood RM, de la Monte S, Convery K, Munzenrider JE, Mirimanoff RO (1992) The role of radiotherapy in the treatment of subtotally resected benign meningiomas. J Neurooncol 13(2): 157–164
34. Nicolato A, Foroni R, Alessandrini F, Bricolo A, Gerosa M (2002) Radiosurgical treatment of cavernous sinus meningiomas" experience with 122 treated patients. Neurosurgery 51: 1153–1161
35. Niiro M, Yatsushiro K, Nakamura K, Kwahara Y, Kuratsu J (2000) Natural history of elderly patients with asymptomatic meningiomas. J Neurol Neurosurg Psychiatry 68: 25–28
36. Novotny J Jr, Novotny J, Vymazal J *et al* (1998) Assessment of the accuracy of stereotactic target localization using magnetic resonance imaging: a phantom study. J Radiosurgery 1: 99–111
37. Olivero WC, Lister JR, Elwood PW (1995) The natural history and growth rate of asymptomatic meningiomas: a review of 60 patients. J Neurosurg 83: 222–224
38. O'Sullivan MG, Loveren HR, Tew JM (1997) The surgical resectability of meningiomas of the cavernous sinus. Neurosurgery 40: 238–247
39. Pan DH, Guo WY, Chang YC *et al* (1998) The effectiveness and factors related to treatment results of gamma knife radiosurgery of meningiomas. Stereotact Funct Neurosurg 70 [Suppl] 1: 19–32
40. Pendl G, Schrottner O, Eustacchio S, Feichtinger K, Ganz J (1997) Stereotactic radiosurgery of skull base meningiomas. Minim Invas Neurosurg 40: 87–90
41. Roche PH, Regis J, Dufour H *et al* (2000) Gamma knife radiosurgery in the management of cavernous sinus meningiomas. J Neurosurg 93 [Suppl] 3: 68–73
42. Samii M, Tatagiba M (1992) Experience with 36 surgical cases of petroclival meningiomas. Acta Neurochirurg (Wien) 118(1–2): 27–32
43. Samii M, Tatagiba M, Monteiro ML (1996) Meningiomas involving the parasellar region. Acta Neurochir (Wien) [Suppl] 65: 63–65
44. Samii M, Carvalho GA, Tatagiba M, Matthies C (1997) Surgical management of meningiomas originating in Meckel's cave. Neurosurgery 41(4): 767–775
45. Sekhar LN, Jannetta PJ, Burkhart LE, Janosky JE (1990) Meningiomas involving the clivus: a six-year experience with 41 patients. Neurosurgery 27(5): 764–781
46. Sekhar LN, Altschuler EM (1991) Meningiomas of the cavernous sinus. In: Al-Mefty O (ed) Meningiomas. Raven Press, New York, pp 445–460
47. Shin M, Kurita H, Sasaki T *et al* (2001) Analysis of treatment outcome after stereotactic radiosurgery for cavernous sinus meningiomas. J Neurosurg 95(3): 435–439
48. Sindou MP, Alaywan M (1998) Most intracranial meningiomas are not cleavable tumors: anatomic-surgical evidence and angiographic predictability. Neurosurgery 42: 476–480
49. Steiner L, Prasad D, Lindquist Ch, Steiner M (1997) Clinical aspects of gamma knife stereotactic radiosurgery. In: Gildenberg P , Tasker R (eds) Textbook of stereotactic and functional neurosurgery. McGraw-Hill, New York, pp 772–774
50. Subach BR, Lunsford LD, Kondziolka D, Maitz AH, Flickinger JC (1998) Management of petroclival meningiomas by stereotactic radiosurgery. Neurosurgery 42(3): 437–445
51. Tamiya T, Ono Y, Matsumoto K, Ohmoto T (2001) Peritumoral brain edema in intracranial meningiomas: effects of radiological and histological factors. Neurosurgery 49: 1046–1052
52. Tanaka T, Kobayashi T, Kida Z (1996) Growth control of cranial base meningiomas by stereotactic radiosurgery with a Leksell Gamma Knife unit. Neurol Med Chir 36(1): 7–10
53. Tishler RB, Loeffler JS, Lunsford LD *et al* (1993) Tolerance of cranial nerves of the cavernous sinus to radiosurgery. Int J Radiation Oncology Biol Phys 27: 215–221
54. Van Havenbergh T, Carvalho G, Tatagiba M, Plets Ch, Samii M (2003) Natural history of petroclival meningiomas. Neurosurgery 52: 55–64
55. Wilson BC (1994) Meningiomas: genetics, malignancy, and the role of radiation in induction and treatment. J Neurosurg 81: 666–675
56. Yamashita J, Handa H, Iwaki K, Abe M (1980) Recurrence of intracranial meningiomas, with special reference to radiotherapy. Surg Neurol 14: 33–40
57. Yasargil MG (1996) Microneurosurgery of CNS tumors. Georg Thieme Verlag, New York, pp 134–185
58. Yoneoka Y, Fujii Y, Tanaka R (2000) Growth of incidental meningiomas. Acta Neurochir (Wien) 42: 507–511
59. Zentner J, Meyer B, Vieweg U, Herberhold C, Schramm J (1997) Petroclival meningiomas: is radical resection always the best option? J Neurol Neurosurg Psychiatry 62(4): 341–345
60. Zevgaridis D, Medele RJ, Muller A, Hischa AC, Steiger HJ (2001) Meningiomas of the sellar region presenting with visual impairment: impact of various prognostic factors on surgical outcome in 62 patients. Acta Neurochir (Wien) 143(5): 471–476

Correspondence: Roman Liščák, M.D., Ph.D., Hospital Na Homolce, Roentgenova 2, Prague 150 30, Czech Republic. e-mail: roman.liscak@homolka.cz

Acta Neurochir (2004) [Suppl] 91: 75–78

Results of outpatient gamma knife radiosurgery for primary therapy of acoustic neuromas

A. Muacevic[1], **A. Jess-Hempen**[1], **J. C. Tonn**[2], and **B. Wowra**[1]

[1] German Gamma Knife Center Munich, Ludwig-Maximilians University, Munich, Germany
[2] Department of Neurosurgery, Ludwig-Maximilians University, Munich, Germany

Summary

Stereotactic radiosurgery (SRS) has been recognized as a non-invasive alternative to surgery for the treatment of acoustic neuromas. Purpose of the current study was to define the impact of outpatient gamma knife radiosurgery (GKS) for patients with unilateral sporadic acoustic neuromas treated within ten years. Follow-up images were analyzed using tumor volume measurements. 219 patients with sporadic acoustic neuromas were treated by GKS as primary therapy. Patients with NF-2 tumors were excluded. Patients were eligible for GKS up to a size limit of 12.5 cm^3. The median follow up time was 6 years after radiosurgery. The local tumor control rate was high (97%). Cranial nerve morbidities were comparably low. 10% of the patients developed hearing loss after radiosurgery and one patient experienced a transient facial neuropathy (0.5%). Transient trigeminal neuropathy developed in 12 patients (5%) and was found to be dependent on the tumor size before treatment. Outpatient gamma knife radiosurgery is a safe and effective treatment method for selected patients with sporadic vestibular schwannomas.

Keywords: Gamma knife; radiosurgery; vestibular schwannoma; acoustic neurinoma.

Introduction

Acoustic neuroma, also known as vestibular schwannoma, is a benign tumor arising from Schwann cells, which comprise the myelin sheath of the vestibulocochlear nerve (CN VIII). It usually arises from the vestibular portion of the nerve and can be located inside the internal acoustic meatus or the cerebellopontine angle, or it can have both intracanalicular and cerebellopontine angle components. The majority of acoustic neuromas grow slowly but ultimately require intervention [25]. The traditional management for acoustic neuroma is surgical excision, however, gamma knife radiosurgery is becoming increasingly relevant as an alternative to microsurgical tumor resection as it combines an effective and safe minimal-invasive treatment and the possibility to perform it on an outpatient basis. With radiosurgery the long term tumor control rates and cranial nerve morbidity appear comparable to those after surgery. We report the impact of gamma knife radiosurgery for 219 patients with unilateral sporadic vestibular schwannomas treated within 10 years by outpatient gamma knife surgery performed in a single institution with respect to tumor growth control, hearing preservation, and the rate of facial and trigeminal neuropathy.

Material and methods

219 patients were treated bei outpatient GKS between October 1994 and October 2002 in our institution. Tumor volume was classified according to the Hannover classification for the extent of tumor growth [22]. Conventional fractionated radiotherapy was not applied. Follow-up stereotactic MR imaging was performed by placing the patient's head into the localizer box of the Leksell stereotactic system, which was coupled to the Leksell stereotactic base frame. In contrast to the treatment procedure, the frame was not rigidly fixed to the patient's skull for the follow-up examinations. Identical MR imaging sequences, however, were used for both the follow-up studies and for the treatment planning. An MR imager (Expert 1.0 tesla; Siemens, Erlangen, Germany) was used for all examinations. To check for MR image distortions, all patients were also examined with computer tomography (HigQ; Siemens) for treatment planning but not for follow-up examination. The first clinical and imaging follow-up examination after GKS was performed after 6 months. Afterwards, patient follow-up examinations were done once every year. These follow-up examinations included an MR imaging volumetric analysis and pure tone audiograms for acoustic function testing. Pre- and postoperative acoustic function was analyzed with the Hannover classification system (steps of 30 dB for the audiometric classification) (Table 1) [21].

Table 1. *Hearing function before radiosurgery according to the Hannover classification*

Audiometric hearing classification	Number of patients	Percentage
1	11	5%
2	42	19%
3	46	21%
4	30	14%
5	90	41%
	219	100%

Table 2. *Hearing function 6 months after radiosurgery according to the Hannover classification*

Audiometric hearing classification	Number of patients	Percentage
1	7	3%
2	19	9%
3	31	14%
4	50	23%
5	112	51%
	219	100%

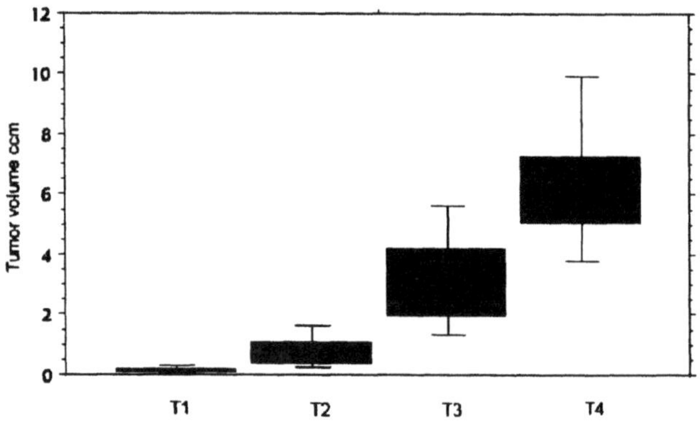

Fig. 1. Is depicting the tumor volume before radiosurgery according to the Hannover classification

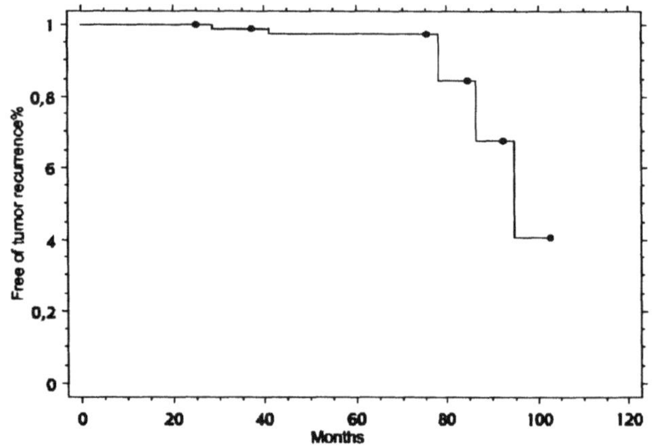

Fig. 2. Is showing the tumor recurrence rate after gamma knife radiosurgery. Five years after radiosurgery the recurrence free survival rate was 97%

Results

The median follow-up period was six years (range 2–10 years). Tumor volume was from 0.1 cm^3 to 10.1 cm^3 (Fig. 1). The actuarial recurrence-free survival was 97% after 5 years (Fig. 2). Six patients experienced a local tumor recurrence. Four of these patients were sucessfully treated by additional gamma knife radiosurgery, two patients underwent surgery. The median dose to the tumor margin was 13 Gy (range 10–15 Gy). The median isodose was 50% (range 40–85%). A mean of six isocenters (range 1–23) were used for radiosurgical treatment. New transient facial neuropathy developed in one patient after radiosurgery (0.5%). Most patients had hearing deficits before radiosurgery. The hearing function was reduced in all classes of the Hannover classification system six months after radiosurgery (Table 2). In seven out of the eleven patients without hearing deficits before radiosurgery the hearing function could be preserved. 10% of the patients developed hearing loss after radiosurgery. Hearing loss was not correlated to the tumor size before treatment. New trigeminal neuropathy developed in 12 patients. This symptom was significantly correlated to the size of the tumor before radiosurgery ($p = 0.007$). 40% of the patients showed a tumor swelling between 4 and 9 months (mean 7 months) after radiosurgery. The mean tumor volume increase was 120% of the initial size. No patient experienced hydrocephalus, vagal or glossopharyngeal nerve dysfunction, or cerebellar signs.

Discussion

Microsurgery and radiosurgery are alternative and complementary modalities to treat acoustic neuromas [19, 20, 23, 26]. Modern microneurosurgery techniques (operating microscope, magnetic resonance imaging (MRI), cranial nerve monitoring) have significantly decreased morbidity and mortality [21, 22, 24], but recent literature also reflects the application and refinement of stereotactic radiosurgery techniques [3–5, 7, 10, 13, 16]. The goals of both microsurgery and radiosurgery are now preservation of facial nerve function and, when feasible, hearing preservation [17, 18, 21].

One should compare only the most recent results of microsurgery and radiosurgery because there has been improvement over the years in both techniques. Both treatment modalities have established a correlation between tumor size and associated treatment-related morbidity, but radiosurgery series have demonstrated markedly diminished cranial and noncranial nerve morbidities, even for larger tumors [9]. Matthies and Samii reported their microsurgical results after acoustic neuroma surgery. 979 of 1000 tumors were totally removed. The recurrence rate was 0.7%. The acute facial paresis rate was 45% and other major neurological complications occurred in approximately 6% of the patients. The rate of hearing preservation was 39.5%. During the early gamma knife experience in the second half of the 1980s, the incidence of facial neuropathy was also high. Flickinger *et al.* reported facial neuropathy in 33% and trigeminal neuropathy in 37% of patients treated with the gamma knife [2]. A subsequent study by the same author analysed 190 patients treated with contemporary radiosurgical technique and reduced tumor dose. The median follow up was 30 months and the median marginal tumor dose was 13 Gy. Our results are remarkably consistent with those reported by Flickinger *et al.*. The 5-year tumor control rate was virtually the same as in our analysis (97%). In the subset of patients who received <15 Gy no new onset of facial weakness was reported [6]. The gradual lowering of the prescribed radiation dose to these tumors, however, almost eliminated the incidence of neuropathies nowadays. The mean dose used in our series was also 13 Gy which seems to be appropriate for both a high tumor control rate and a low complication rate. Only one patient experienced a transient facial neuropathy after gamma knife treatment. This outcome compares favorably with results after fractionated stereotactic and conventional fractionated radiotherapy [1, 8, 11, 12, 17, 25]. New trigeminal neuropathy developed in 12 patients after radiosurgery. Interestingly, this symptom was significantly correlated to the size of the tumor before gamma knife radiosurgery ($p = 0.007$). Once the tumor was shrinking the symptom also diminished.

Radiosurgery has been shown to achieve local tumor control rates comparable to total microsurgical resection. However, with the tumor remaining in situ the goal of therapeutic results has to be redefined. Local control is contributed to tumors that show volume reduction or stable tumor volume following radiosurgery [27]. Some authors claim the ongoing debate about the uncertainty of long term tumor control may be obsolete since major studies have shown that tumor recurrences are unlikely after more than three years following radiosurgical treatment [9]. This statement should be regarded cautiously as four of the six recurrent tumors developed five years after treatment in the current study.

Transient tumor swelling is a widely recognized phenomenon and is usually associated with loss of central enhancement [28]. Yu *et al.* found a transient increase in tumor volume in 57 out of 126 acoustic neuromas with a peak at 6 months after sequential tumor volume mapping. In the current study 40% of the patients experienced a tumor swelling after radiosurgery. The mean increase in volume swelling was 120% of the initial tumor volume with a peak 7 months after therapy. Obviously, transient swelling has significant clinical implications, particularly when larger tumors are treated. Patients and referring physicians must be educated in advance about the possibility of transient swelling and its effects. In this regard patients may be wrongly advised to undergo open surgery during the swelling period. Patience may be all that is required.

In the current study MR imaging was performed in all patients as a basic imaging modality for treatment planning. High resolution MR imaging enhances tumor volume definition and facilitates more sophisticated treatment plans using greater numbers of isocenters and the use of lower treatment doses. These changes are well documented in the literature. MR imaging resulted in a significant reduction in cranial neuropathies after radiosurgery [3, 14, 15].

Conclusions

Based on the results presented herein for tumor control, facial nerve function, and hearing preservation, radiosurgery can be offered as a safe alternative primary treatment modality for acoustic neuromas of suitable size, regardless of the patient's medical status.

References

1. Andrews DW, Silverman CL, Glass J *et al* (1995) Preservation of cranial nerve function after treatment of acoustic neurinomas with fractionated stereotactic radiotherapy. Preliminary observations in 26 patients. Stereotact Funct Neurosurg 64: 165–182
2. Flickinger JC, Lunsford LD, Linskey ME *et al* (1993) Gamma

knife radiosurgery for acoustic tumors: Multivariate analysis of four year results. Radiother Oncol 27: 91–98
3. Flickinger JC, Kondziolka D, Pollock BE *et al* (1996) Evolution in technique for vestibular schwannoma radiosurgery and effect on outcome. Int J Radiat Oncol Biol Phys 36: 275–280
4. Flickinger JC, Kondziolka D, Lunsford LD (1996) Dose and diameter relationships for facial, trigeminal, and acoustic neuropathies following acoustic neuroma radiosurgery. Radiother Oncol 41: 215–219
5. Flickinger JC, Niranjen A, Kondziolka D *et al* (1999) Current results of acoustic neuroma radiosurgery: Years 5–10 of the University of Pittsburgh experience. Int J Radiat Oncol Biol Phys 45 [Suppl] 1: 171–172
6. Flickinger JC, Kondziolka A, Niranjan *et al* (2001) Results of acoustic neuroma radiosurgery: an analysis of 5 years' experience using current methods. J Neurosurg 94: 1–6
7. Foote RL, Coffey RJ, Swanson JW (1995) Stereotactic radiosurgery using the gamma knife for acoustic neuromas. Int J Radiat Oncol Biol Phys 32: 1153–1160
8. Kagei K, Shirato H, Suzuki K *et al* (1999) Small-field fractionated radiotherapy with or without stereotactic boost for vestibular schwannoma. Radiother Oncol 50: 341–347
9. Kondziolka D, Lunsford LD, McLaughlin MR *et al* (1998) Long-term outcomes after radiosurgery for acoustic neuromas. N Engl J Med 339: 1426–1433
10. Koos WT, Matula C, Levy D *et al* (1995) Microsurgery versus radiosurgery in the treatment of small acoustic neurinomas. Acta Neurochir (Wien) [Suppl] 63: 73–80
11. Maire JP, Caudry M, Darrouzet V *et al* (1995) Fractionated radiation therapy in the treatment of stage III and IV cerebellopontine angle neurinomas: Long-term results in 24 cases. Int J Radiat Oncol Biol Phys 32: 1137–1143
12. Marks LB (1993) Conventional fractionated radiation therapy vs. radiosurgery for selected benign intracranial lesions (arteriovenous malformations, pituitary adenomas, and acoustic neuromas). J Neurooncol 17: 223–230
13. Mendenhall WM, Friedman WA, Bova FJ (1994) Linear accelerator-based stereotactic radiosurgery for acoustic schwannomas. Int J Radiat Oncol Biol Phys 28: 803–810
14. Miller RC, Foote RL, Coffey RJ *et al* (1999) Decrease in cranial nerve complications after radiosurgery for acoustic neuromas: A prospective study of dose and volume. Int J Radiat Oncol Biol Phys 43: 305–311
15. Niranjan A, Lunsford LD, Flickinger JC *et al* (1999) Dose reduction improves hearing preservation rates after intracanalicular acoustic tumor radiosurgery. Neurosurgery 45: 753–762
16. Ogunrinde OK, Lunsford LD, Flickinger JC (1994) Stereotactic radiosurgery for acoustic nerve tumors in patients with useful preoperative hearing: Results at 2-year follow-up examination. J Neurosurg 80: 1011–1017
17. Poen J, Golby A, Forster A (1999) Fractionated stereotactic radiosurgery and preservation of hearing in patients with vestibular schwannoma: a preliminary report. Neurosurgery 45: 1299–1307
18. Pollock BE, Kondziolka D, Flickinger JC *et al* (1993) Preservation of cranial nerve function after radiosurgery for nonacoustic schwannomas. Neurosurgery 33: 597–601
19. Pollock BE, Lunsford LD, Kondziolka D (1995) Outcome analysis of acoustic neuroma management: A comparison of microsurgery and stereotactic radiosurgery. Neurosurgery 36: 215–224
20. Pollock BE, Lunsford LD, Kondziolka D (1998) Vestibular schwannoma management. Part II. Failed radiosurgery and the role of delayed microsurgery. J Neurosurg 89: 949–955
21. Samii M, Matthies C (1997) Management of 1000 vestibular schwannomas (acoustic neuromas): hearing function in 1000 tumor resections. Neurosurgery 40: 248–260
22. Samii M, Matthies C (1997) Management of 1000 vestibular schwannomas (acoustic neuromas): the facial nerve – preservation and restitution of function. Neurosurgery 40: 684–694
23. Sekhar LN, Gormley WB, Wright DC (1996) The best treatment for vestibular schwannoma (acoustic neuroma): Microsurgery or radiosurgery? Am J Otol 17: 676–682
24. Tonn JC, Schlake HP, Goldbrunner R *et al* (2000) Acoustic neuroma surgery as an interdisciplinary approach: a neurosurgical series of 508 patients. J Neurol Neurosurg Psychiatry 69: 161–166
25. Varlotto JM, Shrieve DC, Alexander E 3rd *et al* (1996) Fractionated stereotactic radiotherapy for the treatment of acoustic neuromas: preliminary results. Int J Radiat Oncol Biol Phys 36: 141–145
26. Yamakami I, Uchino Y, Kobayashi E *et al* (2003) Conservative management, gamma-knife radiosurgery, and microsurgery for acoustic neuromas: a systematic review of outcome and risk of three therapeutic options. Neurol Res 25: 682–690
27. Yamamoto M, Jimbo M, Ide M *et al* (1999) Is unchanged tumor volume after radiosurgery a measure of outcome? Stereotact Funct Neurosurg 66: 231–239
28. Yu CP, Cheung JY, Leung S (2000) Sequential volume mapping for confirmation of negative growth in vestibular schwannomas treated by gamma knife radiosurgery. J Neurosurg 93 [Suppl] 3: 82–89

Correspondence: Alexander Muacevic, M.D., German Gamma Knife Center, Ingolstädterstr. 166, 80939 Munich, Germany. e-mail: Alexander.Muacevic@med.uni-muenchen.de

Acta Neurochir (2004) [Suppl] 91: 79–87

Gamma knife radiosurgery for patients with multiple cerebral metastases

B. E. Lippitz[1], **T. Kraepelien**[1], **K. Hautanen**[1], **M. Ritzling**[1], **T. Rähn**[2], **E. Ulfarsson**[2], and **J. Boethius**[2]

[1] Gamma Knife Center, H.M. Queen Sophia Hospital (Sophiahemmet), Stockholm, Sweden
[2] Department of Neurosurgery and Gamma Knife, Karolinska University Hospital, Stockholm, Sweden

Summary

Although efficacy of gamma knife radiosurgery has been demonstrated in numerous studies, the policies in patients with multiple metastases seem to be unequivocal. The maintained quality of life, the possibility of short hospitalization and the continuation of a systemic chemotherapy are increasingly important arguments in favor of a minimally invasive radiosurgical approach. These factors are particularly emphasized in patients with a dismal prognosis.

The current retrospective analysis was undertaken to summarize the clinical results of radiosurgery in patients with multiple cerebral metastases of various primary cancer. Fractionated whole brain radiotherapy (WBRT) was omitted as prophylactic treatment and applied only in cases with general tumor spread. Clinical data of all consecutive patients (n = 215) who received gamma knife radiosurgery for cerebral metastases between January 2001 and January 2003 at the gamma knife Centers of the Karolinska Hospital and H.M. Queen Sophia Hospital (Sophiahemmet) Stockholm were analyzed retrospectively. 172 patients were treated for multiple metastases (198 treatments).

The median prescription dose was 22 Gy (range 14–34 Gy). The Kaplan Meier plot shows a median survival (MST) of 7.8 months for patients with multiple cerebral metastases and 13.7 months for patients with single metastases. There was no relation between survival and number of metastases in patients with multiple metastases. Within this group 11.6% (20/172 patients) developed adverse radiation reactions. Tumor recurrences were documented by FDG-PET in 7 patients (out of 172 patients: 4.1%) after a median latency of 10 months after radiosurgery.

In summary, gamma knife radiosurgery provides a highly effective and minimally invasive method to treat patients with multiple cerebral metastases even without prophylactic WBRT. Local control and patient survival in the present series of patients is in accordance with other retrospective series of patients with single and multiple metastases.

Keywords: Multiple metastases; cerebral metastases; radiosurgery; minimally invasive.

Introduction

The need, possibilities and necessity for palliative treatment for patients with cerebral metastases are important issues in the discussion between patients, providers of care and insurance companies in Europe. The effect and invasiveness of the local treatment of brain metastases has gained importance with increasing progress of the systemic oncological treatment regimens. Statistics indicate that about 400 patients per million people are presenting with brain metastases every year, and yet there is no general strategy dealing with this situation. The treatment policies vary particularly for patients with multiple cerebral metastases. The therapy decision depends often on regional preferences, varying between fractionated whole brain fractionated radiotherapy (WBRT), multiple resections, radiosurgery with either Linac or gamma knife or in some instances supportive care only.

A meaningful surgical resection is not achievable in the majority of patients with multiple brain metastases. A common alternative option is the treatment with conventional whole brain radiotherapy. Series after fractionated radiotherapy of multiple cerebral metastases, however report a relatively low efficacy with median survival times (MST) between 2.9 [20] and 4.2 months [7]. The negative prognosis for patients with cerebral metastases treated with WBRT has influenced even selection and indication for the systemic therapies of the primary cancer. Generally chemotherapy is interrupted during WBRT and eventually even an operation for a primary cancer may no longer be considered indicated in the presence of brain metastases. With radiosurgery potentially being able to control the cerebral disease, the implication on chemotherapy and other systemic regimens may change and a more aggressive approach can be provided without interruption during treatment of the brain tumors.

So far more than 80.000 patients with cerebral metastases have been treated world-wide using gamma knifes. Both local tumor control and survival appear favorable in radiosurgical series when compared to studies after conventional radiotherapy. In Stockholm fractionated whole brain radiotherapy is administered only in patients with general cerebral tumor spreading or after open tumor resection. All other patients are treated with gamma knife only, since numerous retrospective studies documented that the omission of WBRT did not affect the prognosis for radiosurgically treated patients with cerebral metastases.

The current retrospective analysis was undertaken in order to summarize the radiosurgical treatment results in a consecutive series of non-selected patients with multiple metastases. The results are specifically analyzed with regard to survival and potential radiosurgery related side-effects.

Patients and methods

Clinical data of all patients who received gamma knife radiosurgery for cerebral metastases between January 2001 until January 2003 at the two gamma knife Centers of the Karolinska Hospital and H.M. Queen Sophia Hospital (Sophiahemmet) in Stockholm were analyzed retrospectively. The final follow-up was obtained in March 2004.

Patient selection

Patients with one to seven cerebral metastases with an individual size of less than 12 cc were accepted for gamma knife Radiosurgery. Between 10/2001 and 10/2003 215 patients were treated at the gamma knife Centers of the Karolinska University Hospital and the H.M. Queen Sophia Hospital in Stockholm. 172 patients were treated for multiple metastases; 645 metastases were treated; 43 patients underwent radiosurgery for single metastases. A median of 3 metastases (range 2–11) was present in patients with multiple tumors. The median age was 63 years (range 31–90 years) in patients with multiple metastases. Among patients with multiple metastases were 44% (n = 76) with lung cancer, 21% (n = 36) with malignant melanoma, 11% (n = 19) with mammary cancer, 9% with renal cancer and 4% (n = 7) with colon cancer. Fractionated radiotherapy of cerebral metastases was only used in patients with a general tumor spread not manageable with radiosurgery. This policy has been described earlier [9]. Patients who developed further tumors after initial radiosurgery were treated with several sessions of radiosurgery for multiple tumors and were summarized in the group of multiple metastases. Therefore a total of 241 treatments were carried out among 215 patients; 15% of patients with multiple metastases were treated again for further metastases. The median prescription dose was 22 Gy (range 14–34 Gy). Generally a prescription isodose between 40% and 60% was chosen depending on the ideal conformity of the prescribed dose. Tumor volumes ranged between 0.04 and 24.7 cc (median 0.6 cc). Karnofsky status was not taken into consideration among selection criteria. Patients with tumors larger than 12 cc were generally declined and referred to microsurgery unless considered inoperable.

Statistical method

The survival was analyzed with the Kaplan Meier Actuarial method using the Log Rank test to determine significant differences among categories of patients.

Radiation reaction

A radiation reaction or alternatively tumor recurrence was considered in case of secondary increase of edema and ultimately increasing contrast enhancement around the treated target. In case of increasing contrast enhancement an FDG-PET-study was performed to differentiate between a potential tumor recurrence and radiation reaction. An increased uptake in FDG-PET was interpreted as increased metabolism indicating a local tumor recurrence.

Results

Survival

The Kaplan Meier plot shows a median survival time (MST) of 7.8 months for patients with multiple cerebral metastases (n = 172). Patients with single metastases showed a median survival of 13.7 months (Fig. 1). Differences were not statistically significant (Log Rank Test 0.079). Within the group of patients with multiple cerebral metastases there were 14.5% (25 patients) who survived less than 2 months. Seventy-nine patients (45.9%) survived more than 9 months, 55 patients with multiple metastases survived more than 10 months (31.9%) (Fig. 3). Tumor recurrences were documented by FDG-PET in 7 patients (out of 172 patients: 4.1%). Local recurrences appeared after a median of 10 months (range 5–21 months). One patient had been treated with a low peripheral dose of 14 Gy and experienced an early tumor recurrence 5 months after radiosurgery. There was no relation between survival and number of metastases in patients with multiple metastases (Fig. 2).

Adverse radiation effects

Within the group of patients with multiple metastases 11.6% (20 patients) developed adverse radiation reactions with secondary increasing edema and eventually contrast enhancement. Generally these patients were differentiated from tumor recurrences by FDG-PET scan. 20.2% of patients with multiple metastases with documented survival of more than 9 months (16 out of 79) experienced an adverse radiation reaction. There was no specific histological group with a higher chance for the development of side effects.

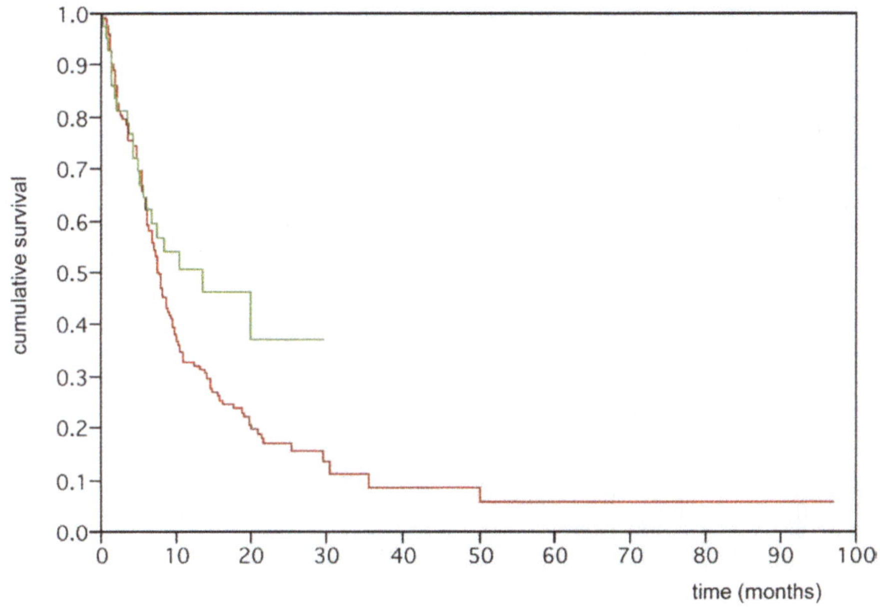

Fig. 1. Kaplan Meier survival plot of patients with single metastases (green line): MST of 13.7 months and patients with multiple metastases (red line): MST 7.8 months (Log Rank Test 0.079)

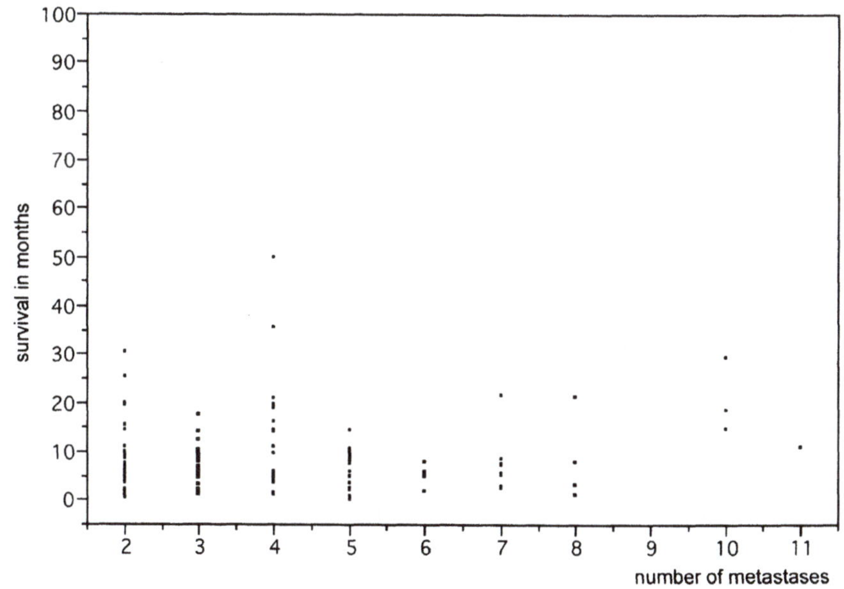

Fig. 2. Number of metastases vs. survival in months for patients with multiple metastases. The number of metastases had no predictive value

Discussion

The current study documents the survival of patients with multiple cerebral metastases of various primary cancers after treatment with gamma knife radiosurgery. Patients with multiple cerebral metastases survived 7.8 months (MST), patients with single metastases survived 13.7 months (MST). The cohort of patients was only minimally selected according to clinical criteria without emphasis on Karnofsky performance status, a fact reflected by the percentage of patients surviving less than 2 months (14.5%). The group of patients with a particularly negative prognosis and a resulting survival of less than 2 months can by definition not be influenced by radiosurgery due to the inherent latency of the method and thereby the time

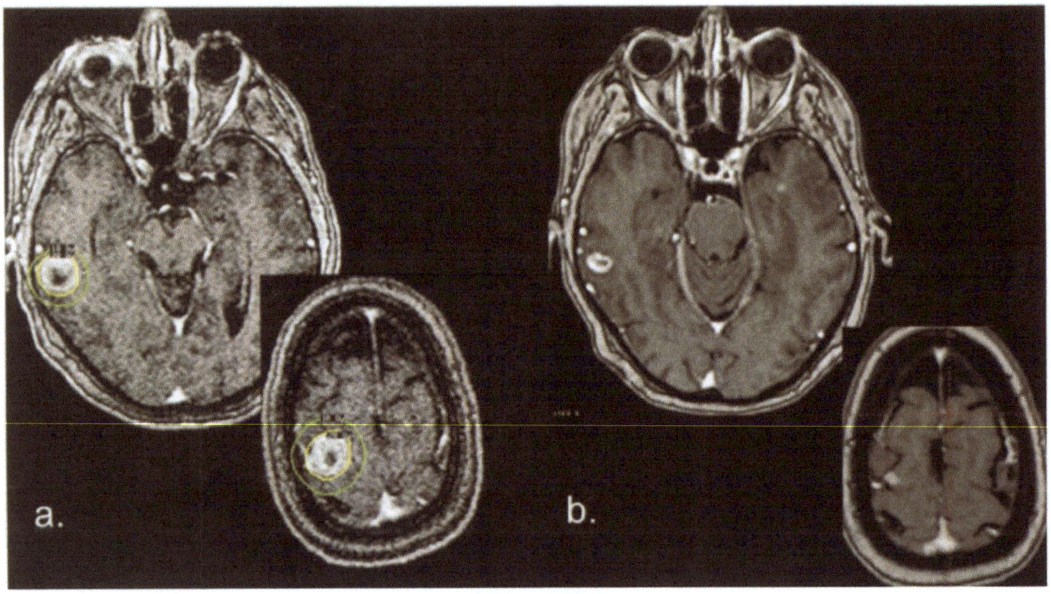

Fig. 3. Patient with multiple cerebral metastases of lung cancer (*NSCLC*) treated with Gamma Knife radiosurgery alone. (a) MRI with contrast enhancement at Gamma Knife treatment. (b) Follow-up study 10 months after radiosurgery. The image documents the typical tumor volume reduction with a minor remaining contrast enhancement

required for a radiosurgically induced volume reduction. No major mass relief and therefore clinical benefit can be expected within less than 2 months. In these terminally ill patients radiosurgery has obviously not provided any effect and the initial selection criteria might have to be questioned. The identification and prediction of these terminally ill patients, however is difficult and does not always follow criteria as defined by RPA classes [7]. In all other patients with a life expectancy of more than 2 months (n = 147), radiosurgery provided an effective palliation with only very low morbidity and more than 53.7% (79/147) surviving more than 9 months.

Annually in Sweden about 4300 patients per 1 million present with cancer (ca. 39.000 patients); according to conservative estimates about 8.5% of cancer patients will develop cerebral metastases [29]. Limited treatment options remain after the diagnosis of multiple brain metastases. Untreated patients have a median survival time (MST) of less than 7 weeks [3].

Only single groups favor an aggressive approach with multiple resections and conventional radiotherapy [25, 28]. One prerequisite to qualify for this invasive approach is a good clinical condition and generally a controlled primary cancer. A likewise invasive therapeutic regimen combining open surgery and fractionated whole brain radiotherapy has been summarized in a recent series [28]. The survival rate in this aggressive treatment regimen was almost identical when compared to the current minimally invasive approach with gamma knife radiosurgery: the surgical resection combined with WBRT in patients with single cerebral metastasis resulted in a MST of 13 months [28]. A retrospective analysis from the Mayo clinic showed that no patient from a radiosurgical group experienced a local recurrence whereas 58% of patients who had been treated by surgery alone had local failure [23]. The difference was statistically significant. Therefore WBRT is generally recommended after a surgical resection to avoid local recurrences. Only when surgical resection is combined with fractionated WBRT the local control seems to be as effective as in the minimal invasive radiosurgical approach using the Gamma knife [18].

Standard treatment for patients with multiple brain metastases includes steroid medication and external beam whole brain irradiation (WBRT). The results are generally disappointing, but the treatment is still widely applied (in Sweden: annually about 110 patients per million). The presence of multiple cerebral metastases is generally associated with a dismal prognosis and affects even the selection, timing and the general indications for the systemic cancer treatment in a negative manner.

The results of fractionated whole brain radiation therapy for cerebral metastases have been summarized in a retrospective analysis of several RTOG studies including 1200 patients. Eighty percent of patients were summarized in RPA classes II and III with a median survival of less than 4.2 months [7]. Another recent retrospective study of patients with brain metastases treated with conventional fractionated radiotherapy revealed a median survival of 2.9 months (528 patients) [20]. Likewise a median survival of 4 months was reported in a series of patients with multiple cerebral metastases treated with conventional radiotherapy alone [21]. A large German retrospective study with 916 patients who had been operated and treated with fractionated WBRT showed a median survival of 3.4 months [15]. The subgroup of older patients (> 65 y) with multiple brain metastases (and uncontrolled primary cancer) survived only 1.2 months with conventional radiotherapy [15]. Median survival from presentation with brain metastases to death was 3 months in another series of 345 patients with multifocal disease [22].

These large retrospective studies demonstrate the limited effect of fractionated radiotherapy for patients with cerebral metastases and a particularly negative prognosis for patients with multiple metastases or older patients. Furthermore, the fractionated radiotherapy involves a lengthy hospitalization plus potential side effects thereby affecting the patient's quality of life. With regard to the limited prognosis, efforts must be made to increase the efficacy of the treatment and to reduce hospitalization and treatment time. Generally systemic chemotherapy is interrupted during conventional radiotherapy of cerebral metastases. In case of gamma knife radiosurgery, a longer interruption is not necessary, which may affect the general prognosis in a positive manner. Radiosurgery with gamma knife or stereotactic linear accelerator generally requires a very short hospitalization and fulfills the requirements of increased efficacy as shown in numerous retrospective studies.

Although the number of patients with multiple metastases treated with radiosurgery is increasing, very few studies have addressed multiple metastases separately. A recently published series compared the outcome of patients with multiple metastases after radiosurgery or WBRT in a retrospective analysis: the patients in the radiosurgical group had a documented MST of 12.5 months (377 days). The group of patients who had received only WBRT only survived 6.6 months (MST: 199 days). The difference was statistically significant [32]. A European gamma knife study demonstrated a median survival of 6 months and a local control in 94% in a series of 97 patients with 97 patients with a median of 3 metastases [31].

Comparable in sample size and primary cancer, two independent retrospective analyses demonstrate the efficacy of gamma knife radiosurgery: A group of 70 patients with multiple cerebral metastases of renal carcinoma was treated with fractionated WBRT resulting in a MST of 3 months [40]. A second independent series of 75 patients with multiple metastases of renal carcinoma were treated with repeated gamma knife treatment with a reported MST of 11.1 months [39].

Selection criteria as defined in RPA classes are crucial in prediction of survival [7, 11]. One of the few prospective randomized studies compared the effects of a radiosurgical boost in patients with multiple brain metastases. Treatment with WBRT alone resulted in local failure at 1 year in 100%. Boost radiosurgery increased the local control considerably resulting in only 8% local failures. The median time to local failure was 6 months after WBRT alone in comparison to 36 months after WBRT plus radiosurgery ($p = 0.0005$) [12, 13]. A recent study of breast cancer metastases treated with gamma knife demonstrated a very typical local tumor control: 94% of patients did not experience local brain tumor recurrence after single session radiosurgery [19]. These results are highly reproducible and have been reported in numerous studies. The summary of 20 retrospective studies dealing with local control and survival of combined 3033 patients with cerebral metastases treated with radiosurgery provided very consistent and reproducible results with reported median survival times between 7.5 and 12 months and local tumor control between 71 and 97 percent (Table 1) [1, 4, 6, 8, 10, 14, 16–19, 24, 26, 27, 30, 33–39].

The survival of patients with multiple metastases in the present study was similar to the mentioned radiosurgical series that describe the outcome in the treatment of various cancer types in mixed groups with single and multiple brain metastases. The present study documented the efficacy of gamma knife Radiosurgery for patients with multiple metastases with a median survival of 7.8 months. Patients with single brain metastases even reached a median survival of 13.7 months. The increased survival reflects a more benign clinical course, since none of these patients developed further metastases during the follow-up, whereas 15% of patients with multiple metastases presented with distant new tumors. It must be considered

Table 1. *Summary of recent publications after radiosurgical treatment of brain metastases*

Study	Number of patients	Local control %	Survival (months)	
Gerosa M, Briccolo A *et al* [8] Stereotact Funct Neurosurg 1996	225	88.0	9.3	various cancer
Shiau CY, Larson DA *et al* [35] Int J Radiat Oncol Biol Phys 1997	100	77.0	12	various cancer
Kim YS, Lunsford LD *et al* [10] Cancer 1997	77	85.0	10	lung carcinoma (NSCLC)
Wowra B, Czempiel H *et al* [39] Radiologe 1997	126	89.5	11.8	various cancer
Mori Y, Lunsford LD *et al* [17] Int J Radiat Oncol Biol Phys 1998	60	88.4	7	melanoma
Mori Y, Lunsford LD *et al* [16] Cancer 1998	35	90.0	11	renal cell carcinoma
Seung SK, Larson DA *et al* [33] Cancer J Sci Am 1998	55	89.0	8.8	melanoma
Chen JC, Apuzzo ML *et al* [4] Stereotact Funct Neurosurg 1999	190	89.0	8.5	various cancer
Muacevic A, Reulen HJ *et al* [18] J Neurosurg 1999	56	83.0	8.8	various cancer
Sneed PK, Larson DA *et al* [37] Int J Radiat Oncol Biol Phys 1999	105	71.0 (radiosurgery alone)	11	various cancer
Lavine SD, Apuzzo ML *et al* [14] Neurosurgery 1999	45	97.0	8	melanoma
Sansur CA, Eisenberg H *et al* [27] Stereotact Funct Neurosurg 2000	173	82.0	7.5	various primary
Amendola BE, Bloch L *et al* [1] Cancer J 2000	68	94.0	7.8	breast cancer
Simonova G, Novotny J *et al* [36] Radiother Oncol 2000	237	91.1		various primary solitary
Schöggl A, Ungersbock K *et al* [30] Acta Neurochir (Wien) 2000	67	95.0	12	various primary
Firlik KS, Lunsford LD *et al* [6] Ann Surg Oncol 2000	30	93.0	13	breast cancer
Petrovich Z, Apuzzo ML *et al* [24] J Neurosurg 2002	458		9	various primary
Sheehan JP, Lunsford LD *et al* [34] J Neurosurg 2002	273	84.0	10 (adenoca.) 7 (other NSCLC)	lung cancer
Sanghavi SN, Mehta MP *et al* [26] Int J Radiat Oncol Biol Phys 2001	502		10.7	various primary
Muacevic A, Wowra B [19] Cancer 2004	151	94.0	10	breast cancer

relevant for the future selection of patients for radiosurgery that the present study could not establish a predictive prognostic value for the number of metastases in patients with multiple tumors.

A multi-institutional study with 502 patients compared the results of a radiosurgical boost applied in combination with WBRT in comparison with the effects of WBRT alone. The evaluation showed a clear advantage for the addition of radiosurgery boost, resulting in a median survival of 16.1 months for the best prognostic group (RPA I) and 10.7 months for the entire series [26].

The recently published RTOG study 9508 has not found the same efficacy of radiosurgery in the treatment of multiple brain metastases after fractionated whole brain radiotherapy, but stated significant differences of survival for patients with solitary metastases and for younger patients with an advantage for radiosurgically treated patients [2]. The survival of patients with multiple metastases in this prospective study was reported with 5.8 months and was thereby shorter than in our retrospective analysis (7.8 months). This fact is interesting, since the RTOG study only analyzed patients in the more favorable prognostic classes and

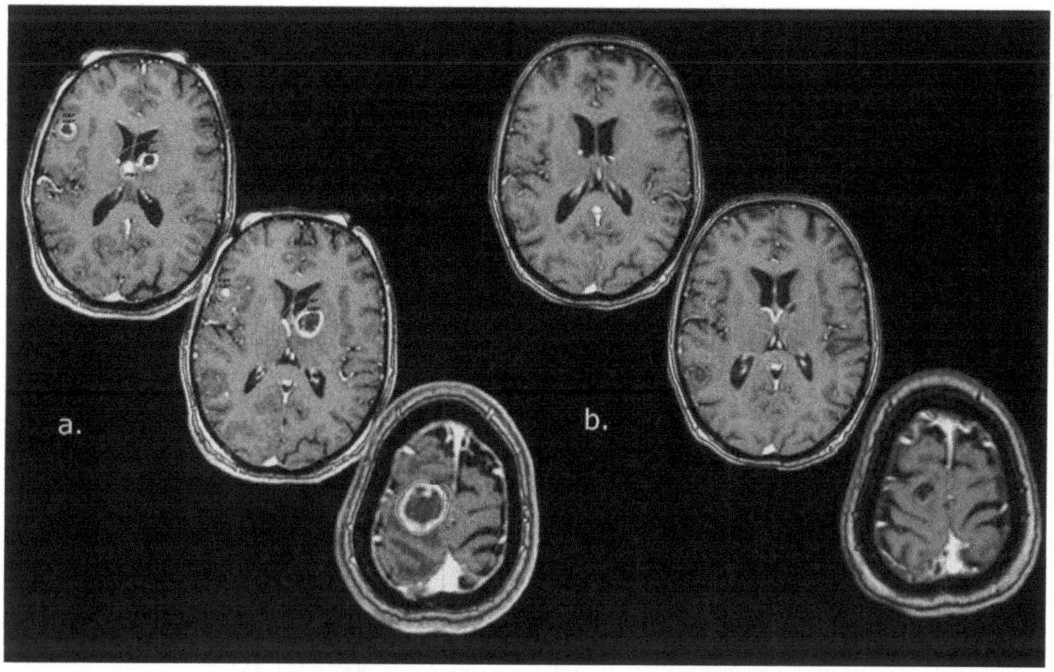

Fig. 4. Patient with breast cancer and multiple cerebral metastases (n = 18). Combination of Gamma Knife radiosurgery for the larger and critically located tumors (prescription dose 19 Gy) with conventional fractionated radiotherapy (*WBRT*) due to general tumor spreading. (a) MRI with contrast enhancement at Gamma Knife treatment. (b) Follow-up three months later. The patient has not developed any neurological symptoms

excluded patients within the worst prognostic class (RPA III). All of the radiosurgical retrospective analyses cited above report longer survival [1, 4, 6, 8, 10, 14, 16–19, 24, 26, 27, 30, 33–38]. Additionally the RTOG result may have been influenced by the fact that the randomized analysis included 19% of patients within the radiosurgical group who never received radiosurgery. Some of these patients who had died or had declined further treatment before the planned radiosurgery was carried out, were still evaluated within the radiosurgical cohort.

A very important finding of this prospective randomized study [2], however, was the statement that patients in the stereotactic radiosurgery group were more likely to have a stable or improved Karnofsky Performance Status (KPS) at 6 months follow-up when compared to patients after fractionated radiotherapy alone. This aspect of improved quality of life related to radiosurgery has been increasingly focused in recent years. Whole brain radiotherapy is still applied in the majority of patients with multiple cerebral metastases. No study however, has so far been able to document a survival benefit for the application of fractionated radiotherapy when compared to stereotactic radiosurgery. The retrospective analyses and the mentioned prospective studies document both a more favorable prognosis and increased quality of life for the minimally invasive approach using radiosurgery.

The current strategy for Swedish patients with brain metastases does not include prophylactic whole brain radiotherapy. Potential distant new metastases are treated with multiple gamma knife sessions. WBRT was applied only in cases with a more general tumor spread (Fig. 4). The length of survival in our series supports this regimen, which seems clearly beneficial when compared to other reports after whole brain fractionated radiotherapy [7, 15, 20–22]. Multiple radiosurgical sessions are considered less invasive and require only a short hospitalization. The strategy has been reported earlier for renal cell carcinoma [9, 39]. A similar protocol was used in a recent publication from the Cleveland clinic showing the most beneficial prognosis for patients where WBRT was postponed and used in cases of general progression [5].

Without affecting prognosis and survival, the rate of new cerebral metastases seems to be reduced when WBRT is applied [5]. So far, there is no significant evidence that fractionated WBRT increases either local control or survival. Several recent studies comprising more than 950 radiosurgically treated patients have not documented any differences in survival or local tumor control when fractionated whole brain radiotherapy was omitted [4, 5, 17, 37].

In summary, gamma knife radiosurgery provides a highly effective method to treat patients with multiple cerebral metastases. Local control and patient survival in the present series of patients is in accordance with other retrospective series of patients with single and multiple metastases. The risk for adverse radiation effects or local recurrences was low when the described selection criteria concerning dose and maximal tumor volume were applied. Combination with WBRT does not seem to influence local control or survival, but can be safely applied when needed in case of a more general tumor spread.

References

1. Amendola BE, Wolf AL, Coy SR, Amendola M, Bloch L (2000) Gamma knife radiosurgery in the treatment of patients with single and multiple brain metastases from carcinoma of the breast. Cancer J 6(2): 88–92
2. Andrews DW, Scott CB, Sperduto PW, Flanders AE, Gaspar LE, Schell MC, Werner-Wasik M, Demas W, Ryu J, Bahary JP, Souhami L, Rotman M, Mehta MP, Curran WJ Jr (2004) Whole brain radiation therapy with or without stereotactic radiosurgery boost for patients with one to three brain metastases: phase III results of the RTOG 9508 randomised trial. Lancet 363(9422): 1665–1672
3. Cairncross JG, Kim JH, Posner JB (1980) Radiation therapy for brain metastases. Ann Neurol 7: 529–541
4. Chen JC, O'Day S, Morton D, Essner R, Cohen-Gadol A, MacPherson D, Giannotta SL, Petrovich Z, Yu C, Apuzzo ML (1999) Stereotactic radiosurgery in the treatment of metastatic disease to the brain. Stereotact Funct Neurosurg 73(1–4): 60–63
5. Chidel MA, Suh JH, Reddy CA, Chao ST, Lundbeck MF, Barnett GH (2000) Application of recursive partitioning analysis and evaluation of the use of whole brain radiation among patients treated with stereotactic radiosurgery for newly diagnosed brain metastases. Int J Radiat Oncol Biol Phys 47(4): 993–999
6. Firlik KS, Kondziolka D, Flickinger JC, Lunsford LD (2000) Stereotactic radiosurgery for brain metastases from breast cancer. Ann Surg Oncol 7(5): 333–338
7. Gaspar L, Scott C, Rotman M, Asbell S, Phillips T, Wasserman T, McKenna WG, Byhardt R (1997) Recursive partitioning analysis (RPA) of prognostic factors in three Radiation Therapy Oncology Group (RTOG) brain metastases trials. Int J Radiat Oncol Biol Phys 37(4): 745–751
8. Gerosa M, Nicolato A, Severi F, Ferraresi P, Masotto B, Barone G, Foroni R, Piovan E, Pasoli A, Bricolo A (1996) Gamma knife radiosurgery for intracranial metastases: from local tumor control to increased survival. Stereotact Funct Neurosurg 66 [Suppl] 1: 184–192
9. Karlsson B, Wersäll P, Lippitz B, Kihlström L (2000) Repeated radiosurgery versus fractionated radiotherapy in the treatment of brain metastases from renal cancer. In: Kondziolka D (ed) Radiosurgery 1999. Karger, Basel, vol 3, pp 232–239
10. Kim YS, Kondziolka D, Flickinger JC, Lunsford LD (1997) Stereotactic radiosurgery for patients with nonsmall cell lung carcinoma metastatic to the brain. Cancer 80(11): 2075–2083
11. Kim DG, Chung HT, Gwak HS, Paek SH, Jung HW, Han D (2000) Gamma knife radiosurgery for brain metastases: prognostic factors for survival and local control. J Neurosurg 93 [Suppl] 3: 23–29
12. Kondziolka D, Patel A, Lunsford LD, Kassam A, Flickinger JC (1999) Stereotactic radiosurgery plus whole brain radiotherapy versus radiotherapy alone for patients with multiple brain metastases. Int J Radiat Oncol Biol Phys 45(2): 427–434
13. Kondziolka D, Lunsford LD, Flickinger JC (2001) Controversies in the management of multiple brain metastases: the roles of radiosurgery and radiation therapy. Forum (Genova) 11(1): 47–58
14. Lavine SD, Petrovich Z, Cohen-Gadol AA, Masri LS, Morton DL, O'Day SJ, Essner R, Zelman V, Yu C, Luxton G, Apuzzo ML (1999) Gamma knife radiosurgery for metastatic melanoma: an analysis of survival, outcome, and complications. Neurosurgery 44(1): 59–64; discussion 64–66
15. Lutterbach J, Bartelt S, Stancu E, Guttenberger R (2002) Patients with brain metastases: hope for recursive partitioning analysis (RPA) class 3. Radiother Oncol 63(3): 339–345
16. Mori Y, Kondziolka D, Flickinger JC, Logan T, Lunsford LD (1998) Stereotactic radiosurgery for brain metastasis from renal cell carcinoma. Cancer 83(2): 344–353
17. Mori Y, Kondziolka D, Flickinger JC, Kirkwood JM, Agarwala S, Lunsford LD (1998) Stereotactic radiosurgery for cerebral metastatic melanoma: factors affecting local disease control and survival. Int J Radiat Oncol Biol Phys 42(3): 581–589
18. Muacevic A, Kreth FW, Horstmann GA, Schmid-Elsaesser R, Wowra B, Steiger HJ, Reulen HJ (1999) Surgery and radiotherapy compared with gamma knife radiosurgery in the treatment of solitary cerebral metastases of small diameter. J Neurosurg 91(1): 35–43
19. Muacevic A, Kreth FW, Tonn JC, Wowra B (2004) Stereotactic radiosurgery for multiple brain metastases from breast carcinoma. Cancer 100(8): 1705–1711
20. Nieder C, Nestle U, Motaref B, Walter K, Niewald M, Schnabel K (2000) Prognostic factors in brain metastases: should patients be selected for aggressive treatment according to recursive partitioning analysis (RPA) classes? Int J Radiat Oncol Biol Phys 46(2): 297–302
21. Nieder C, Andratschke N, Grosu AL, Molls M (2003) Recursive partitioning analysis (RPA) class does not predict survival in patients with four or more brain metastases. Strahlenther Onkol 179(1): 16–20
22. Nussbaum ES, Djalilian HR, Cho KH, Hall WA (1996) Brain metastases. Histology, multiplicity, surgery, and survival. Cancer 78(8): 1781–1788
23. O'Neill BP, Iturria NJ, Link MJ, Pollock BE, Ballman KV, O'Fallon JR (2003) A comparison of surgical resection and stereotactic radiosurgery in the treatment of solitary brain metastases. Int J Radiat Oncol Biol Phys 55(5): 1169–1176
24. Petrovich Z, Yu C, Giannotta SL, O'Day S, Apuzzo ML (2002) Survival and pattern of failure in brain metastasis treated with stereotactic gamma knife radiosurgery. J Neurosurg 97 [Suppl] 5: 499–506
25. Pollock BE, Brown PD, Foote RL, Stafford SL, Schomberg PJ (2003) Properly selected patients with multiple brain metastases may benefit from aggressive treatment of their intracranial disease. J Neurooncol 61(1): 73–80
26. Sanghavi SN, Miranpuri SS, Chappell R, Buatti JM, Sneed PK, Suh JH, Regine WF, Weltman E, King VJ, Goetsch SJ, Breneman JC, Sperduto PW, Scott C, Mabanta S, Mehta MP (2001)

Radiosurgery for patients with brain metastases: a multi-institutional analysis, stratified by the RTOG recursive partitioning analysis method. Int J Radiat Oncol Biol Phys 51(2): 426–434

27. Sansur CA, Chin LS, Ames JW, Banegura AT, Aggarwal S, Ballesteros M, Amin P, Simard JM, Eisenberg H (2000) Gamma knife radiosurgery for the treatment of brain metastases. Stereotact Funct Neurosurg 74(1): 37–51
28. Schackert G, Steinmetz A, Meier U, Sobottka SB (2001) Surgical management of single and multiple brain metastases: results of a retrospective study. Onkologie 24(3): 246–255
29. Schouten LJ, Rutten J, Huveneers HA, Twijnstra A (2002) Incidence of brain metastases in a cohort of patients with carcinoma of the breast, colon, kidney, and lung and melanoma. Cancer 94(10): 2698–2705
30. Schöggl A, Kitz K, Reddy M, Wolfsberger S, Schneider B, Dieckmann K, Ungersbock K (2000) Defining the role of stereotactic radiosurgery versus microsurgery in the treatment of single brain metastases. Acta Neurochir (Wien) 142(6): 621–626
31. Schöggl A, Kitz K, Ertl A, Reddy M, Bavinzski G, Schneider B (1999) Prognostic factor analysis for multiple brain metastases after gamma knife radiosurgery: results in 97 patients. J Neurooncol 42(2): 169–175
32. Serizawa T, Iuchi T, Ono J, Saeki N, Osato K, Odaki M, Ushikubo O, Hirai S, Sato M, Matsuda S (2000) Gamma knife treatment for multiple metastatic brain tumors compared with whole-brain radiation therapy. J Neurosurg 93 [Suppl] 3: 32–36
33. Seung SK, Sneed PK, McDermott MW, Shu HK, Leong SP, Chang S, Petti PL, Smith V, Verhey LJ, Wara WM, Phillips TL, Larson DA (1998) Gamma knife radiosurgery for malignant melanoma brain metastases. Cancer J Sci Am 4(2): 103–109
34. Sheehan JP, Sun MH, Kondziolka D, Flickinger J, Lunsford LD (2002) Radiosurgery for non-small cell lung carcinoma metastatic to the brain: long-term outcomes and prognostic factors influencing patient survival time and local tumor control. J Neurosurg 97(6): 1276–1281
35. Shiau CY, Sneed PK, Shu HK, Lamborn KR, McDermott MW, Chang S, Nowak P, Petti PL, Smith V, Verhey LJ, Ho M, Park E, Wara WM, Gutin PH, Larson DA (1997) Radiosurgery for brain metastases: relationship of dose and pattern of enhancement to local control. Int J Radiat Oncol Biol Phys 37(2): 375–383
36. Simonova G, Liscak R, Novotny J Jr, Novotny J (2000) Solitary brain metastases treated with the Leksell gamma knife: prognostic factors for patients. Radiother Oncol 57(2): 207–213
37. Sneed PK, Lamborn KR, Forstner JM, McDermott MW, Chang S, Park E, Gutin PH, Phillips TL, Wara WM, Larson DA (1999) Radiosurgery for brain metastases: is whole brain radiotherapy necessary? Int J Radiat Oncol Biol Phys 43(3): 549–558
38. Petrovich Z, Yu C, Giannotta SL, O'Day S, Apuzzo ML (2002) Survival and pattern of failure in brain metastasis treated with stereotactic gamma knife radiosurgery. J Neurosurg 97 [Suppl] 5: 499–506
39. Wowra B, Horstmann GA, Cibis R, Czempiel H (1997) Profile of ambulatory radiosurgery with the gamma knife system. 2: report of clinical experiences. Radiologe 37(12): 1003–1015
40. Wowra B, Siebels M, Muacevic A, Kreth FW, Mack A, Hofstetter A (2002) Repeated gamma knife surgery for multiple brain metastases from renal cell carcinoma. J Neurosurg 97(4): 785–793

Correspondence: Bodo Lippitz, Gamma Knife Center, H.M. Queen Sophia Hospital (Sophiahemmet), Valhallavägen 91, 114 86 Stockholm, Sweden. e-mail: bodo.lippitz@sophiahemmet.se

Acta Neurochir (2004) [Suppl] 91: 89–102

Special indications in gamma knife surgery

B. Wowra[1], **A. Muacevic**[1], **S. Müller-Schunk**[1], and **J.-C. Tonn**[2]

[1] German Gamma Knife Centre Munich, Munich, Germany
[2] Department of Neurosurgery, Ludwig-Maximilians University, Munich, Germany

1. Pilocytic astrocytoma

Summary

Pilocytic astrocytoma (PA) represent a rare indication for Gamma Knife Surgery. Mostly small remnants after surgical debulking are treated. The prognosis depends on specific variants of biological and clinical criteria. In this regard we differentiated two groups of tumors; the so-called 'typical' tumors with a histological grading of WHO Grade I, no prior fractionated radiotherapy and no cystic component and the so called 'atypical' tumors with either a malignant transformation, previous fractionated radiotherapy and/or cystic components. The outcome after GKS was much more favourable for typical PA than for atypical. In typical cases a high tumor control with a very low risk of side effects can be achieved.

Keywords: Gamma knife; pilocytic astrocytoma; radiosurgery.

Introduction

Pilocytic astrocytoma is a very rare, generally circumscribed, and usually benign brain tumor occurring in children and young adults. Pilocytic astrocytoma harbour a considerable clinical and biological variation. They produce focal neurological deficits or non-localizing signs. Typically pilocytic astrocytomas maintain their WHO grade I status over years or decades. There are rare cases of pilocytic astrocytomas undergoing malignant transformation. Since most of such tumors had undergone prior conventional radiotherapy, radiation may be a factor promoting malignant change [9].

The present contribution is an attempt to reflect the current position of Gamma Knife Surgery (GKS) in the therapeutic armoury for pilocytic astrocytoma. A review of the literature is given and the results obtained in Munich during a 10-year-period of outpatient GKS are analysed.

Patients and results

Within ten years ten patients received 12 GKS sessions for radiosurgical treatment of PA (Table 1). This represents 0.4% of all GKS procedures in our centre. The reasons for repeated GKS were a "two-fraction" strategy in a patient previously irradiated by conventional radiotherapy and malignant tumor transformation to a grade III tumor, which has been proven histologically in another patient. Median age was 27.5 years (9.5–57.6). All tumors had surgical tumor debulking before GKS. The tumors involved the hypothalamus in three patients, cerebellum in five, as well as the brainstem and thalamus in one patient each. The targets of GKS were small remnants of tumor amounting to a median tumor volume of 1.7 cm^3 (0.4 cm^3–17.0 cm^3). The lesions were treated with a median dose to the tumor margin of 13.8 Gy (10 Gy–18 Gy) corresponding to a peripheral isodose of 50% (50%–70%).

Tumors with a WHO grade higher than I (1 case), with previous fractionated radiotherapy (1 case) or with cystic components (2 cases) were scored as "atypical" pilocytic astrocytomas ($n = 4$). The dose parameters showed no statistical significant difference for typical (6 cases) and atypical tumors (Table 1). One death occurred due to recurrence and malignant tumor transformation to a grade III tumor of the brain stem. Side effects were restricted to cyst formation in one patient and a cyst progression in another case (both received surgical therapy). Time event analysis using Kaplan-Meier statistics showed differences in the outcome of the two biological subtypes of PA (Fig. 1). The patients with typical PA are alive without side effects after GKS. The tumor control rate was 100% for typical PA corresponding to a median survival time of 5.3 years (range 2–7.7). The outcome of atypical tumors was clearly inferior to that but did not reach statistical significance because of the small sample size. Typical PA showed regression of tumor mass after GKS as evidenced by volumetric follow up of the treated radiosurgical target (Fig. 2).

Discussion

Pilocytic astrocytoma is a typical "special indication" of gamma knife surgery because these lesions are very rare. The incidence rate of 4.8 per 1 million per year [7] and their clinical and biological heterogeneity precludes sophisticated prospective therapeutic trials. In our material, the percentage of GKS treatments for

Table 1. *Characteristics and treatment data of ten PA patients treated by GKS*

	All patients	Typical PA	Atypical PA	Significance
Sex				
Male	2	1	1	
Female	8	5	3	
Age (range)	27.5 (9.5–57.6)	18.6 (9.5–37.9)	41.0 (24.5–57.6)	$p < 0.05$
Karnofsky's performance score	90 (70–100)	100 (90–100)	70 (70–80)	$p < 0.01$
Neurol. deficit before GKS	5	2 (40%)	3 (100%)	
Fractionated radiotherapy	1	0	1	
Surgical interventions	1 (1–2)	1 (1–2)	2 (1–2)	
Interval (range)				
1. surgery – GKS (y)	6.1 (0.5–16.9)	6.0 (0.5–16.9)	4.9 (1.1–11.9)	n.s.
Tumor localization				
Thalamus	1	0	1	
Hypothalamus	3	2	1	
Cerebellum	5	4	1	
Pons	1	0	1	
Treatment parameters				
Tumor volume (cm^3)	1.7 (0.4–17.0)	1.8 (0.5–2.5)	1.4 (0.4–17.0)	n.s.
Tumor dose (D_{min}, Gy)	13.8 (10–18)	13.5 (11–17)	13.8 (10–18)	n.s.
No. of isocentres	9 (6–26)	9 (6–16)	13 (6–26)	n.s.
Peripheral isodose (%)	50 (50–70)	50 (50–70)	50 (50–50)	n.s.
Outcome after GKS				
Cyst formation after GKS	2	1	1	
Recurrence after GKS	2	0	2	

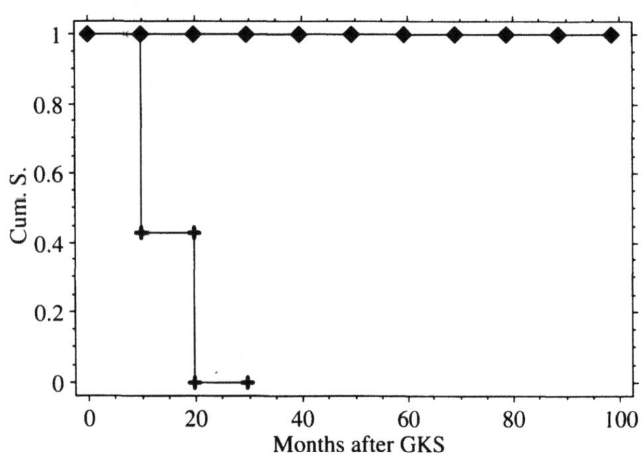

Fig. 1. Tumor control after GKS for typical (rhombs) and atypical (crosses) PA (Kaplan-Meier plot)

pilocytic astrocytoma is 0.4% which is consistent with other series [5, 15, 34].

Astrocytic tumors in general are difficult to treat by a local therapy like radiosurgery because of their infiltrative growth pattern and the absence of a sharp delineation from the surrounding healthy cerebral tissue. In contrast to this, pilocytic astrocytomas are mostly compact and well circumscribed and therefore may represent suitable targets for radiosurgery [34].

Pilocytic astrocytomas have been shown to constitute a distinctive biological subgroup among gliomas [8, 11–13, 16, 19, 20, 27]. They occur mainly in the first two decades of life representing the most common glioma in children. In general, the natural biological behaviour of these tumors is benign [4, 6, 7] but some clinical and biological heterogeneity has been reported in recent years [14, 15]. In some lesions cysts are encountered while other tumors are associated with neurofibromatosis type I [21, 24, 36]. Recently, an atypical variant of pilocytic astrocytoma has been discovered and referred to as pilomyxoid astrocytoma. These tumors are associated with a worse prognosis [22]. In our small cohort of patients, we were able to define two subtypes of pilocytic astrocytoma which showed considerably different outcomes after GKS. This observation corresponds to the data in the recent literature [14, 15, 22] and possibly should be taken into account when deciding on GKS in the future.

Pilocytic astrocytomas may arise in highly eloquent areas of the brain [1, 3, 10, 15, 17, 18, 25, 26, 30–33, 35, 37, 39] and in some patients complete microsurgical resection may be too hazardous [10]. Furthermore, even after uncomplicated surgical resection of cerebellar PA in childhood, a compromised quality of life has been reported [28]. On the other hand, conventional radiation therapy in these tumors is handicapped by frequent recurrences and the risk of mental retardation especially in young children [2, 38]. Inter-

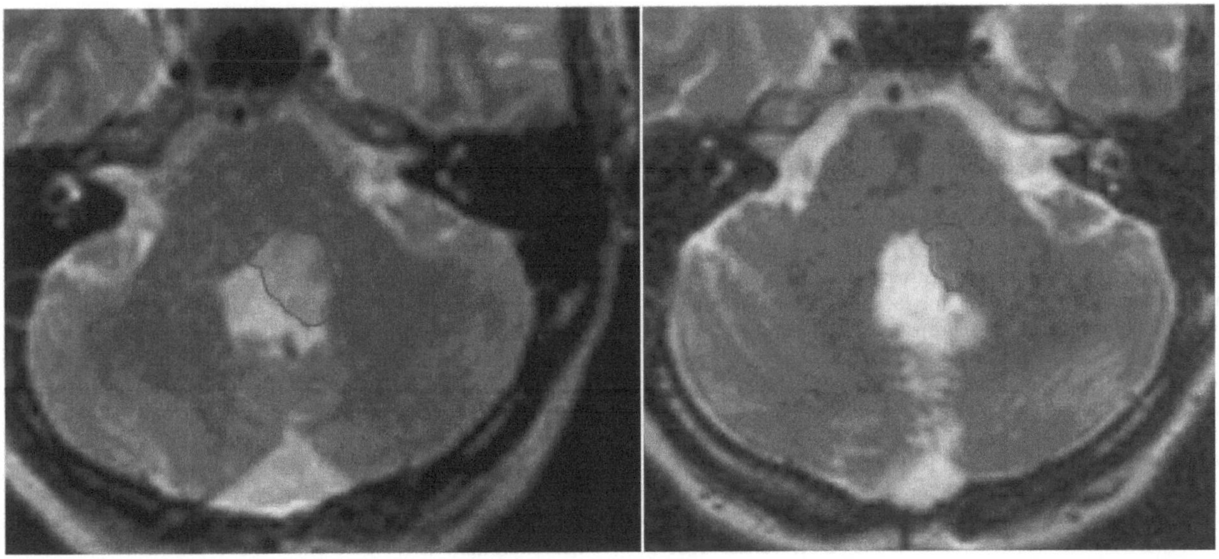

Fig. 2. Residual cerebellar PA after surgical resection. Eight years after GKS the PA decreased from 1.8 cm^3 (left image) to 0.3 cm^3 (right image). No side effects were observed

stitial radiosurgery has been shown to be an alternative to resection of deeply seated pilocytic astrocytomas [23]. In some cystic PA the seed implantation may be supplemented by intracavitary isotope therapy [29]. Interstitial radiosurgery however, may not be feasible in very small lesions located in eloquent anatomical sites and especially in small remnants after subtotal resection. Thus, gamma knife surgery may represent a fourth therapeutic option for non-cystic pilocytic astrocytomas [5, 15, 34]. The prescription doses may be moderate [5] and the documented evidence of GKS for PA reveals a very attractive therapeutic profile particularly in typical cases.

References

1. Amato VG, Arienta C, Sparacio F (1999) Dorsally exophytic brain stem tumors: total removal of a medullary pilocytic astrocytoma in child. Clinicopathological considerations and case report. J Neurosurg Sci 43: 299–304
2. Arita K, Kurisu K, Sugiyama K, Itoh Y, Hotta T, Sogabe T, Uozumi T (2003) Long-term results of conventional treatment of diencephalic pilocytic astrocytoma in infants. Childs Nerv Syst 19: 145–151
3. Barea D, Richez P, Gueguen E, Clavel G, Grisoli F, Briant JF (1999) [Pilocytic astrocytoma of the conus medullaris]. J Radiol 80: 736–738
4. Bernaerts A, Vanhoenacker F, Debois V, Parizel PM (2003) Juvenile pilocytic astrocytoma. Jbr-Btr 86: 142–143
5. Boethius J, Ulfarsson E, Rahn T, Lippitz B (2002) Gamma knife radiosurgery for pilocytic astrocytomas. J Neurosurg 97: 677–680
6. Brown PD, Buckner JC, O'Fallon JR, Iturria NL, Brown CA, O'Neill BP, Scheithauer BW, Dinapoli RP, Arusell RM, Abrams RA, Curran WJ, Shaw EG (2004) Adult patients with supratentorial pilocytic astrocytomas: a prospective multicenter clinical trial. Int J Radiat Oncol Biol Phys 58: 1153–1160
7. Burkhard C, Di Patre PL, Schuler D, Schuler G, Yasargil MG, Yonekawa Y, Lutolf UM, Kleihues P, Ohgaki H (2003) A population-based study of the incidence and survival rates in patients with pilocytic astrocytoma. J Neurosurg 98: 1170–1174
8. Camby I, Nagy N, Lopes MB, Schafer BW, Maurage CA, Ruchoux MM, Murmann P, Pochet R, Heizmann CW, Brotchi J, Salmon I, Kiss R, Decaestecker C (1999) Supratentorial pilocytic astrocytomas, astrocytomas, anaplastic astrocytomas and glioblastomas are characterized by a differential expression of S100 proteins. Brain Pathol 9: 1–19
9. Dirks PB, Jay V, Becker LE, Drake JM, Humphreys RP, Hoffman HJ, Rutka JT (1994) Development of anaplastic changes in low-grade astrocytomas of childhood. Neurosurgery 34: 68–78
10. Fernandez C, Figarella-Branger D, Girard N, Bouvier-Labit C, Gouvernet J, Paz Paredes A, Lena G (2003) Pilocytic astrocytomas in children: prognostic factors – a retrospective study of 80 cases. Neurosurgery 53: 544–553; discussion 554–545
11. Gesundheit B, Klement G, Senger C, Kerbel R, Kieran M, Baruchel S, Becker L (2003) Differences in vasculature between pilocytic and anaplastic astrocytomas of childhood. Med Pediatr Oncol 41: 516–526
12. Giannini C, Scheithauer BW, Burger PC, Christensen MR, Wollan PC, Sebo TJ, Forsyth PA, Hayostek CJ (1999) Cellular proliferation in pilocytic and diffuse astrocytomas. J Neuropathol Exp Neurol 58: 46–53
13. Gutmann DH, Hedrick NM, Li J, Nagarajan R, Perry A, Watson MA (2002) Comparative gene expression profile analysis of neurofibromatosis 1-associated and sporadic pilocytic astrocytomas. Cancer Res 62: 2085–2091
14. Haapasalo H, Sallinen S, Sallinen P, Helen P, Jaaskelainen J, Salmi TT, Paetau A, Paljarvi L, Visakorpi T, Kalimo H (1999)

Clinicopathological correlation of cell proliferation, apoptosis and p53 in cerebellar pilocytic astrocytomas. Neuropathol Appl Neurobiol 25: 134–142
15. Hadjipanayis CG, Kondziolka D, Gardner P, Niranjan A, Dagam S, Flickinger JC, Lunsford LD (2002) Stereotactic radiosurgery for pilocytic astrocytomas when multimodal therapy is necessary. J Neurosurg 97: 56–64
16. Hunter S, Young A, Olson J, Brat DJ, Bowers G, Wilcox JN, Jaye D, Mendrinos S, Neish A (2002) Differential expression between pilocytic and anaplastic astrocytomas: identification of apolipoprotein D as a marker for low-grade, non-infiltrating primary CNS neoplasms. J Neuropathol Exp Neurol 61: 275–281
17. Hwang SL, Huang TY, Chai CY, Howng SL (1998) Hypothalamic juvenile pilocytic astrocytoma presenting with intracerebral hemorrhage. J Formos Med Assoc 97: 784–787
18. Ideguchi M, Nishizaki T, Harada K, Kwak T, Murakami T, Ito H (1998) Pilocytic astrocytoma of the velum interpositum. Neurol Med Chir (Tokyo) 38: 283–286
19. Ishii N, Sawamura Y, Tada M, Daub DM, Janzer RC, Meagher-Villemure M, de Tribolet N, Van Meir EG (1998) Absence of p53 gene mutations in a tumor panel representative of pilocytic astrocytoma diversity using a p53 functional assay. Int J Cancer 76: 797–800
20. Klein R, Roggendorf W (2001) Increased microglia proliferation separates pilocytic astrocytomas from diffuse astrocytomas: a double labeling study. Acta Neuropathol (Berl) 101: 245–248
21. Kluwe L, Hagel C, Tatagiba M, Thomas S, Stavrou D, Ostertag H, von Deimling A, Mautner VF (2001) Loss of NF1 alleles distinguish sporadic from NF1-associated pilocytic astrocytomas. J Neuropathol Exp Neurol 60: 917–920
22. Komotar RJ, Burger PC, Carson BS, Brem H, Olivi A, Goldthwaite PT, Tihan T (2004) Pilocytic and pilomyxoid hypothalamic/chiasmatic astrocytomas. Neurosurgery 54: 72–79; discussion 79–80
23. Kreth FW, Faist M, Warnke PC, Rossner R, Volk B, Ostertag CB (1995) Interstitial radiosurgery of low-grade gliomas. J Neurosurg 82: 418–429
24. Li J, Perry A, James CD, Gutmann DH (2001) Cancer-related gene expression profiles in NF1-associated pilocytic astrocytomas. Neurology 56: 885–890
25. Martin DS, Geller TJ, Falbo S, Pittman T (2000) Exophytic juvenile pilocytic astrocytomas of the posterior fossa. J Child Neurol 15: 262–265
26. Nadvi SS, Ramdial PK (1998) Transient peduncular hallucinations secondary to brain stem compression by a cerebellar pilocytic astrocytoma. Br J Neurosurg 12: 579–581
27. Nakamizo A, Inamura T, Ikezaki K, Yoshimoto K, Inoha S, Mizoguchi M, Amano T, Fukui M (2002) Enhanced apoptosis in pilocytic astrocytoma: a comparative study of apoptosis and proliferation in astrocytic tumors. J Neurooncol 57: 105–114
28. Pompili A, Caperle M, Pace A, Ramazzotti V, Raus L, Jandolo B, Occhipinti E (2002) Quality-of-life assessment in patients who had been surgically treated for cerebellar pilocytic astrocytoma in childhood. J Neurosurg 96: 229–234
29. Proust F, Coche-Dequeant B, Carpentier P, Laquerriere A, Derlon JM, Blond S, Christiaens J, Freger P (1998) [Combination treatment for pilocytic astrocytoma: stereotaxic radiosurgery and endocavitary radiotherapy]. Neurochirurgie 44: 50–54
30. Reis A, Kuzeyli K, Cobanoglu U, Cakir E, Usul H, Sari A (2003) Pilocytic astrocytoma of neurohypophysis. Neuropathology 23: 214–218
31. Sandberg DI, Souweidane MM (1999) Hemifacial spasm caused by a pilocytic astrocytoma of the fourth ventricle. Pediatr Neurol 21: 754–756
32. Shaya MR, Fowler MR, Nanda A (2004) Pilocytic astrocytoma presenting as an intrinsic brainstem tumor: case report and review of the literature. J La State Med Soc 156: 33–36
33. Sim KB, Hong SK (1999) Multicentric juvenile pilocytic astrocytoma occurring primarily in the trigone of the lateral ventricle. Childs Nerv Syst 15: 477–481
34. Somaza SC, Kondziolka D, Lunsford LD, Flickinger JC, Bissonette DJ, Albright AL (1996) Early outcomes after stereotactic radiosurgery for growing pilocytic astrocytomas in children. Pediatr Neurosurg 25: 109–115
35. Tacconi L, Farah JO, Rossi ML, Jeffreys R (1999) Neurohypophyseal pilocytic astrocytoma invading the skull base. Br J Neurosurg 13: 614–617
36. Tada K, Kochi M, Saya H, Kuratsu J, Shiraishi S, Kamiryo T, Shinohima N, Ushio Y (2003) Preliminary observations on genetic alterations in pilocytic astrocytomas associated with neurofibromatosis 1. Neuro-oncol 5: 228–234
37. Takada Y, Ohno K, Tamaki M, Hirakawa K (1999) Cerebellopontine angle pilocytic astrocytoma mimicking acoustic schwannoma. Neuroradiology 41: 949–950
38. Vinchon M, Assaker R, Soto-Ares G, Ruchoux MM, Dhellemmes P (2001) [Cerebellar pilocytic astrocytomas in children. Report of 72 cases]. Neurochirurgie 47: 83–91
39. Yousry I, Muacevic A, Olteanu-Nerbe V, Naidich TP, Yousry TA (2004) Exophytic pilocytic astrocytoma of the brain stem in an adult with encasement of the caudal cranial nerve complex (IX–XII): presurgical anatomical neuroimaging using MRI. Eur Radiol

2. Non-vestibular nerve schwannoma

Summary

Microsurgical resection remains the method of choice for non-vestibular schwannomas. Radiosurgery with the Leksell gamma knife or the stereotactic linear accelerator can be used as an adjunct or alternative method in suitable patients. The therapeutic profile of radiosurgery is characterized by a very high tumor control rate, mostly associated with significant tumor shrinkage. As a rule, specific side effects are mild and transient. Taking into account a common genetic base (e.g. absence of merlin expression) for all schwannomas, one should apply a uniform dose regime to these tumors irrespective of the cranial nerve matrix.

Keyword: Gamma knife surgery; radiosurgery; schwannoma.

Introduction

Although vestibular schwannoma, formerly referred to as acoustic neuroma, represent the majority of cranial nerve schwannomas, similar tumors may develop on other cranial nerves, too. Loss of merlin expression appears to be a universal finding in all schwannomas indicating a common genetic base for these tumors. The merlin protein is a product of the NF2 gene which turned out to act as a tumor suppressor gene [67]. Be-

Table 1. *Patients and treatment characteristics*

	No.	Median	Min.	Max.
Patients/affected nerves	26			
Age (y)		48.5	15.0	75.2
Sex (female/male)	9/17			
Previous surgery	10 (38.5%)			
Fractionated radiotherapy	0			
N. III	1			
N. V	15 (58%)			
N. VI	1			
N. VII	4 (15%)			
N. IX–X	5			
Marginal Dose (D_{min}, Gy)		13.5	9.0	15.0
Peripheral Isodose (%)		50	50	60
Maximal Dose (D_{max}, Gy)		26.0	18	30
Tumor volume (cm^3)		2.70	0.12	13.0

side the frequent vestibular schwannoma, schwannomas of the trigeminal and facial nerve, and schwannomas of the jugular foramen are of particular clinical significance. There are relatively few reports in the literature dealing with Gamma Knife Surgery for non-vestibular schwannoma. This manuscript is an attempt to summarize the current knowledge of this subject. A review of the literature is compared to the results obtained in Munich during a 10 year period of outpatient gamma knife radiosurgery for non-vestibular schwannoma.

Patients and results

A total of 26 patients were treated for non-vestibular schwannoma (NVS) representing 7% of all schwannomas and less than 1% of all Gamma Knife surgery (GKS) procedures in our centre, respectively. In three individuals, NVS was associated with NF II (one trigeminal schwannoma, facial nerve schwannoma and abducens nerve schwannoma, respectively). The characteristics of the patients and treatment parameters are given in Table 1. In summary, one patient had a third nerve schwannoma, 15 patients had a trigeminal neuroma, 4 a facial nerve schwannoma, one an abducens nerve schwannoma, and 5 schwannomas of the jugular foramen. Ten (38.5%) patients were treated for residual or recurrent NVS after previous surgery. Before GKS all tumors showed specific focal neurological deficits. The median tumor volume was 2.7 cm^3 for all NVS. The facial nerve schwannomas were significantly smaller than the trigeminal nerve schwannomas (0.95 cm^3 range: 0.5–4.0 cm^3; versus 3.2 cm^3 range: 0.3–12.0 cm^3). The dose parameters were statistically not different among the different NVS.

Follow-up information was available for all but two patients. Median follow-up was 68.2 months (range 5.3–105.4). One patient with NF II died of unrelated reasons two years after GKS. All treated NVS were controlled by GKS. Two (8%) tumors were controlled after a period of transient swelling. Complete remission of the tumor volume was observed in 8 (33%) patients, tumor shrinkage in 12 (50%) and a stable tumor size in 2 (8%). The median reduction in tumor volume was 40% after 3 years in serial tumor volumetry. Treatment related side effects were observed in 8 patients (33%). In three out of four patients with facial nerve schwannoma the palsy induced by the tumor increased transiently. In five patients with trigeminal schwannoma the neuralgia and/or neuropathy increased (in four of them transiently). One patient had a severe exacerbation of herpes labialis.

Discussion

Mainly due to the wide-spread distribution of magnetic resonance imaging (MRI) [24] the incidence of vestibular schwannoma (VS) during the past three decades is increasing [13, 37, 64]. Today between 12 and 41 new VS cases are diagnosed in developed countries [8, 13, 37, 63, 64]. In the same time frame,

Table 2. *Survey of radiosurgery and stereotactic radiotherapy for NVS. A total of 86 patients have been treated and reported in the literature*

	Pollock* [47]	Muthukumar# [40]	Mabanta [30]	Isono [15]	Zabel [69]	MUNICH
Year	2002	1999	1999	2002	2001	2004
No. of pts	23	17	18	1	13	26
TN	10		7		7	15
FN			2	1		4
JF	12	17	9		3	5
other	1				3	2
Treatment device	GK	GK	LINAC	GK	LINAC	GK
Fractionation	no	no	no	no	yes	no
Dose (Gy)	18	12–18	13.1	12	57.6 (1.8)	13.5
Tumor vol. (ccm)	8.9		5.5		19.8	2.7
Follow-up (years)	3.6	3.5	2.7		2.8	5.7
morbidity	17%		0%		0%	33%
Control rate	96%	94%	100%		100%	100%

Latest report from Pittsburgh [47] including the earlier series of Pollock *et al*, 1993 [48] Huang *et al*, 1999 [14], and 12 patients of the series of Muthukumar# *et al*, 1999 [40].

TN Trigeminal nerve, *FN* facial nerve, *JF* jugular foramen, *GK* gamma knife.

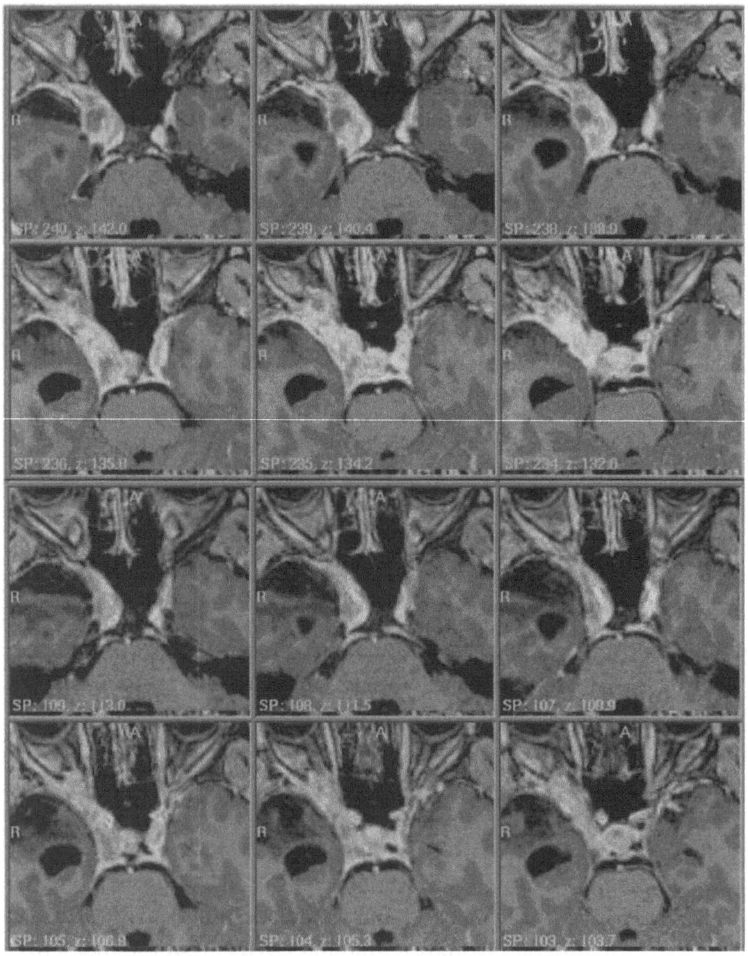

Fig. 1. Follow-up MRI of a patient with a partly resected trigeminal schwannoma. The upper two rows of MRI scans show the tumor before gamma knife radiosurgery. The images in the lower two rows show corresponding scans two years after GKS. The tumor is controlled and considerablly reduced in size

GKS as a minimally invasive alternative to microsurgery for VS has been established [16, 21, 43, 65, 66]. However, schwannomas may also develop with other cranial nerves [1–7, 9–12, 14, 17–19, 23, 25–29, 31–36, 38, 39, 41, 42, 44–46, 49–55, 60–62, 68]. Like in VS, the availability of MRI improved the diagnosis of NVS significantly [51, 56]. Similarly, surgery has been the first line treatment for NVS for five decades. With respect to mortality and morbidity the results of surgery have considerably improved over time [20, 22, 34, 57–59]. The risks of microsurgery are characterized by a low percentage of general morbidity (CSF leakage, hemorrhage etc.) and mostly mild and transient new or increased cranial nerve deficits.

There are a number of treatment reports in the literature reporting treatment results for selected patients with cranial nerve schwannomas treated by either surgery, radiosurgery, fractionated radiotherapy or a combined treatment approach. Kim *et al.* [20], for example, published a surgical series of 18 facial nerve schwannoma. Isono *et al.* [15] treated a case of facial nerve schwannoma by combined surgery and radiosurgery. Schisano *et al.* [59], Konovalov *et al.* [22], and Samii *et al.* [58] published surgical series on trigeminal nerve schwannoma. Huang *et al.* [14] presented a GKS series on trigeminal nerve schwannoma. For schwannomas of the caudal cranial nerves and the foramen jugulare, respectively, Samii *et al.* [57] reported his surgical experience and Zhang *et al.* [70] and Muthukumar *et al.* [40] reported GKS treatment results. Mabanta *et al.* [30] used linear-accelerator technique to treat 18 cases of NVS radiosurgically. Although smaller, his series is similar to ours and the outcome is comparable. Zabel *et al.* [69] treated 13 NVS by stereotactic fractionated radiotherapy with favourable results. Radiosurgery seems to be an effectiv treatment method for selected cases, however, there is a size limit beyond which radiosurgery becomes disadvantageous compared to surgery. In stereotactic fractionated radiotherapy the size of the target lesion is less important when compared to radiosurgery. The draw-back of fractionated radiation therapy is the higher dose load and the much longer treatment time needed as against radiosurgery. Therefore, in selected cases, a combined approach of microsurgery and/or radiosurgery is preferable. This strategy is supported by the available literature (and the current series) where between 37.5% and 76.5% of the radiosurgically treated patients had been operated before. Regarding the specific risk of cranial nerve toxicity, radiosurgery and fractionated radiation therapy are not inferior to surgery taking into account the different tumor sizes.

Apparently, loss of merlin expression constitutes a genetic base common to all schwannomas [67]. Because of this fact, one could theoretically speculate that a similar radiation dose should be appropriate for all schwannomas. Historically, however, a higher dose was applied to NVS than to VS [47]. According to more recently published data [15, 30] and in agreement with our present results a dose level similar to VS should also be appropriate for NVS. Because of radiation protection concerns, the much higher dose delivered with fractionated stereotactic radiation therapy should be restricted to NVS which are not operable and/or too large for gamma knife radiosurgery.

References

1. Anand CS, Kumra PK, Anand TS, Singh SK (1977) Facial nerve schwannoma. J Laryngol Otol 91: 1093–1099
2. Asaoka K, Sawamura Y, Murai H, Satoh M (1999) Schwannoma of the oculomotor nerve: a case report with consideration of the surgical treatment. Neurosurgery 45: 630–634
3. Decrop E, Casselman J, Vandevoorde P, Meeus L (1989) Vagal nerve schwannoma. J Belge Radiol 77: 211
4. Del Priore LV, Miller NR (1989) Trigeminal schwannoma as a cause of chronic, isolated sixth nerve palsy. Am J Ophthalmol 108: 726–729
5. Dinu C, Martu D (1980) [Schwannoma of the facial nerve with intratemporal development]. Rev Chir Oncol Radiol O R L Oftalmol Stomatol Otorinolaringol 25: 107–112
6. Dolan EJ, Tucker WS, Rotenberg D, Chui M (1982) Intracranial hypoglossal schwannoma as an unusual cause of facial nerve palsy. Case report. J Neurosurg 56: 420–423
7. Feinberg AS, Newman NJ (1999) Schwannoma in patients with isolated unilateral trochlear nerve palsy. Am J Ophthalmol 127: 183–188
8. Frohlich AM, Sutherland GR (1993) Epidemiology and clinical features of vestibular schwannoma in Manitoba, Canada. Can J Neurol Sci 20: 126–130
9. Garen PD, Harper CG, Teo C, Johnston IH (1987) Cystic schwannoma of the trochlear nerve mimicking a brain-stem tumor. Case report. J Neurosurg 67: 928–930
10. Ginsberg LE, DeMonte F (1999) Diagnosis please. Case 16: facial nerve schwannoma with middle cranial fossa involvement. Radiology 213: 364–368
11. Gonzales-Pardo L, Brackett CE, Lansky LL (1980) Facial nerve schwannoma in a 16-year-old girl. Childs Brain 7: 220–224
12. Ho KL (1981) Schwannoma of the trochlear nerve. Case report. J Neurosurg 55: 132–135
13. Howitz MF, Johansen C, Tos M, Charabi S, Olsen JH (2000) Incidence of vestibular schwannoma in Denmark, 1977–1995. Am J Otol 21: 690–694
14. Huang CF, Kondziolka D, Flickinger JC, Lunsford LD (1999) Stereotactic radiosurgery for trigeminal schwannomas. Neurosurgery 45: 11–16
15. Isono N, Tamura Y, Kuroiwa T, Nagasawa S, Yamashita M, Tanabe H, Ogawa N (2002) [Combined therapy with surgery and stereotactic radiosurgery for facial schwannoma: case report] No Shinkei Geka 30: 735–739
16. Karpinos M, The BS, Zeck O, Carpenter LS, Phan C, Mai WY, Lu HH, Chiu JK, Butler EB, Gormley WB, Woo SY (2002) Treatment of acoustic neuroma: stereotactic radiosurgery vs. microsurgery. Int J Radiat Oncol Biol Phys 54: 1410–1421
17. Katoh M, Kawamoto T, Ohnishi K, Sawamura Y, Abe H (1999) Asymptomatic schwannoma of the oculomotor nerve: case report. J Clin Neurosci 7: 458–460
18. Kawasaki A (1999) Oculomotor nerve schwannoma associated with ophthalmoplegic migraine. Am J Ophthalmol 128: 658–660
19. Kim CS, Chang SO, Oh SH, Ahn SH, Hwang CH, Lee HJ (2003) Management of intratemporal facial nerve schwannoma. Otol Neurotol 24: 312–316
20. Kim JC, Bhattacharjee M, Amedee RG (2003) Facial nerve schwannoma. Ann Otol Rhinol Laryngol 112: 185–187
21. Kondziolka D, Lunsford LD, McLaughlin MR, Flickinger JC (1998) Long-term outcomes after radiosurgery for acoustic neuromas. N Engl J Med 339: 1426–1433
22. Konovalov AN, Spallone A, Mukhamedjanov DJ, Tcherekajev VA, Makhmudov UB (1996) Trigeminal neurinomas. A series of 111 surgical cases from a single institution. Acta Neurochir (Wien) 138: 1027–1035
23. Koyye RT, Mahadevan A, Santosh V, Chickabasaviah YT, Govindappa SS, Hedge T, Shankar SK (2003) A rare case of cellular schwannoma involving the trigeminal ganglion. Brain Tumor Pathol 20: 79–83
24. Kwan TL, Tang KW, Pak KK, Cheung JY (2004) Screening for vestibular schwannoma by magnetic resonance imaging: analysis of 1821 patients. Hong Kong Med J 10: 38–43
25. Lanzieri CF (1997) Head and neck case of the day. Schwannoma of the right facial nerve. AJR Am J Roentgenol 169: 275, 278–279
26. Lee KS, Britton BH, Kelly DL Jr (2000) Schwannoma of the facial nerve in the cerebellopontine angle presenting with hearing loss. Surg Neurol 32: 231–234
27. Lingawi SS (2000) Oculomotor nerve schwannoma: MRI appearance. Clin Imaging 24: 86–88
28. Lo PA, Harper CG, Besser M (2001) Intracavernous schwannoma of the abducens nerve: a review of the clinical features, radiology and pathology of an unusual case. J Clin Neurosci 8: 357–360

29. Lunardi P, Missori P, Gagliardi FM, Fraioli B (1989) Trigeminal schwannoma with infratemporal extension. Case report. J Neurosurg Sci 33: 293–295
30. Mabanta SR, Buatti JM, Friedman WA, Meeks SL, Mendenhall WM, Bova FJ (1999) Linear accelerator radiosurgery for nonacoustic schwannomas. Int J Radiat Oncol Biol Phys 43: 545–548
31. Mariniello G, Horvat A, Dolenc VV (1999) En bloc resection of an intracavernous oculomotor nerve schwannoma and grafting of the oculomotor nerve with sural nerve. Case report and review of the literature. J Neurosurg 91: 1045–1049
32. Mascarenhas L, Magalhaes Z, Honavar M, Romao H, Resende M, Resende Pereira J, Rocha Vaz (2004) Schwannoma of the abducens nerve in the cavernous sinus. Acta Neurochir (Wien) 146: 389–392
33. Matsui T, Morikawa E, Morimoto T, Asano T (2002) Presigmoid transpetrosal approach for the treatment of a large trochlear nerve schwannoma – case report. Neurol Med Chir (Tokyo) 42: 31–35
34. McCormick PC, Bello JA, Post KD (1990) Trigeminal schwannoma. Surgical series of 14 cases with review of the literature. J Neurosurg 69: 850–860
35. Mehta VS, Singh RV, Misra NK, Choudhary C (1990) Schwannoma of the oculomotor nerve. Br J Neurosurg 4: 69–72
36. Mendez JC, Saucedo G, Melendez B (2004) Cystic trigeminal schwannoma with fluid-fluid levels. Eur Radiol
37. Mirz F, Pedersen CB, Fiirgaard B, Lundorf E (2000) Incidence and growth pattern of vestibular schwannomas in a Danish county, 1977–98. Acta Otolaryngol Suppl 543: 30–33
38. Morrissey MS, Sellars SL (1990) Vagal nerve schwannoma – a new diagnostic sign. Postgrad Med J 66: 42–43
39. Murakami M, Tsukahara T, Hatano T, Nakakuki T, Ogino E, Aoyama T (2004) Olfactory groove schwannoma – case report. Neurol Med Chir (Tokyo) 44: 191–194
40. Muthukumar N, Kondziolka D, Lunsford LD, Flickinger JC (1999) Stereotactic radiosurgery for jugular foramen schwannomas. Surg Neurol 52: 172–179
41. Nakamura M, Carvalho GA, Samii M (2002) Abducens nerve schwannoma: a case report and review of the literature. Surg Neurol 57: 183–189
42. Netuka D, Benes V (2003) Oculomotor nerve schwannoma. Br J Neurosurg 17: 168–173
43. Noren G (1998) Long term complications following gamma knife radiosurgery of vestibular schwannomas. Stereotact Funct Neurosurg 70 [Suppl] 1: 65–73
44. Osterhus DR, Van Loveren HR, Friedman RA (1999) Trigeminal schwannoma. Am J Otol 20: 551–552
45. Pearman K, Welch AR (1980) Schwannoma of the intratemporal facial nerve. Case report J Laryngol Otol 94: 779–784
46. Peco MT, Palacios E (1959) Intracranial and intratemporal facial nerve schwannoma. Ear Nose Throat J 81: 312
47. Pollock BE, Foote RL, Stafford SL (2002) Stereotactic radiosurgery: the preferred management for patients with nonvestibular schwannomas? Int J Radiat Oncol Biol Phys 52: 1002–1007
48. Pollock BE, Kondziolka D, Flickinger JC, Maitz A, Lunsford LD (1993) Preservation of cranial nerve function after radiosurgery for nonacoustic schwannomas. Neurosurgery 33: 597–601
49. Pou JW (1959) Neurinoma (schwannoma) of the facial nerve: report of two cases. AMA Arch Otolaryngol 69: 48–56
50. Radford R, Haigh PM, MacDermott N, Leatherbarrow B (1999) A case of trigeminal schwannoma presenting as Raeder's syndrome in a child. Eye 13(Pt 5): 680–682
51. Rigamonti D, Spetzler RF, Shetter A, Drayer BP (1987) Magnetic resonance imaging and trigeminal schwannoma. Surg Neurol 28: 67–70
52. Rocchi G, Artico M, Lunardi P, Gagliardi FM (1991) Intracranial schwannoma of the facial nerve: report of two cases and review of the literature. Neurochirurgia (Stuttg) 34: 180–183
53. Ross DL, Tew JM Jr, Benton C, Eisentrout C (1984) Trigeminal schwannoma in a child. Neurosurgery 15: 108–110
54. Rubin DI, Matsumoto JY, Suarez GA, Auger RG (1999) Facial trigeminal synkinesis associated with a trigeminal schwannoma. Neurology 53: 635–637
55. Saada AA, Limb CJ, Long DM, Nikarpo JK (2000) Intracanalicular schwannoma of the facial nerve: a manifestation of neurofibromatosis type 2. Arch Otolaryngol Head Neck Surg 126: 547–549
56. Saito A, Nakazawa T, Matsuda M, Handa J (1989) [Comparison of computed tomographic scanning and magnetic resonance imaging in the diagnosis of trigeminal schwannoma. Report of four cases] Neurol Med Chir (Tokyo) 29: 1101–1106
57. Samii M, Babu RP, Tatagiba M, Sepehrnia A (1995) Surgical treatment of jugular foramen schwannomas. J Neurosurg 82: 924–932
58. Samii M, Migliori MM, Tatagiba M, Babu R (1995) Surgical treatment of trigeminal schwannomas. J Neurosurg 82: 711–718
59. Schidano G, Olivecrona H (1960) Neurinomas of the Gasserian ganglion and trigeminal root. J Neurosurg 17: 306–322
60. Shenouda EF, Ghosh A, Coakham HB (2002) Trochlear nerve schwannoma removed by combined petrosal approach. Br J Neurosurg 16: 600–604
61. Steinhart H, Wigand ME, Fahlbusch R, Triebswetter F, Gress H, Iro H [Facial nerve schwannoma in the inner auditory canal and geniculate ganglion] HNO 51: 640–645
62. Tew JM Jr, Yeh HS, Miller GW, Shahbabian S (1983) Intratemporal schwannoma of the facial nerve. Neurosurgery 13: 186–188
63. Tos M, Charabi S, Thomsen J (1997) Increase of diagnosed vestibular schwannoma in Denmark. Acta Otolaryngol Suppl 529: 53–55
64. Tos M, Stangerup SE, Caye-Thomasen P, Tos T, Thomsen J (2004) What is the real incidence of vestibular schwannoma? Arch Otolaryngol Head Neck Surg 130: 216–220
65. Ture U, Ozduman K, Elmaci I, Pamir MN (2002) Infratentorial lateral supracerebellar approach for trochlear nerve schwannoma. J Clin Neurosci 9: 595–598
66. Unger F, Walch C, Papaefthymiou G, Eustachio S, Feichtinger K, Quehenberger F, Pendl G (2002) Long term results of radiosurgery for vestibular schwannomas. Zentralbl Neurochir 63: 52–58
67. Woordruff JM, Kourea HP, Louis DN (1997) Schwannoma. In: Kleihues P, Cavenee WK (eds) Pathology and Genetics of Tumours of the Nervous system, pp. 126–132. Lyon: International Agency for Research on Cancer
68. Yokota N, Yokoyama T, Nishizawa S (1999) Facial nerve schwannoma in the cerebellopontine cistern. Findings on high resolution CT and MR cisternography. Br J Neurosurg 13: 512–515
69. Zabel A, Debus J, Thilmann C, Schlegel W, Wannenmacher M (2001) Management of benign cranial nonacoustic schwannomas by fractionated stereotactic radiotherapy. Int J Cancer 96: 356–362
70. Zhang N, Pan L, Dai JZ, Wang BJ, Wang EM, Cai PW (2002) Gamma knife radiosurgery for jugular foramen schwannomas. J Neurosurg 97: 456–458

3. Capillary cerebellar haemangioblastoma

Summary

This paper summarises the current knowledge of gamma knife radiosurgery for cerebellar haemangioblastomas. A review of the literature is compared to the results obtained in Munich during a 10-year-period of outpatient GKS. We have treated a total of 23 haemangioblastomas in eleven patients with 17 GKS sessions. Median age was 47 years (range 17–59). Two patients had sporadic haemangioblastomas, nine von Hippel-Lindau syndrome. All but one treated tumors did shrink or stopped growing after radiosurgery. Adjoining cysts did not respond to radiosurgery. In one patient a new cyst developed after radiosurgery. Stereotactic radiosurgery is a valuable alternative therapeutic procedure for primary or adjuvant treatment of solid capillary cerebellar haemangioblastoma.

Keywords: Gamma knife surgery; von Hippel-Lindau disease; cerebellar haemangioblastoma.

Introduction

Capillary cerebellar haemangioblastomas are rare tumors. They account for 1–2.5% of all intracranial tumors and 7–12% of all posterior fossa tumors [7, 9]. At diagnosis, they are of very variable size and may have a solid or cystic appearance. They present either as sporadic forms or as manifestation of the von Hippel-Lindau syndrome (VHL). In the latter case, multiple cerebellar haemangioblastomas may be associated with angiomas of the retina and other viscera, with renal cancer and pheochromocytoma [9]. The incidence of VHL is approximately 25 cases per million inhabitants [6, 7]. This hereditary cancer syndrome is caused by germ-line mutations of the VHL tumor suppressor gene. A gene product (referred to as the VHL protein) has been identified and found to have several distinct functions. [13, 15]. According to a French series, the main causes of mortality of VHL are the following: cerebellar haemangioblastomas, renal cancer and pheochromocytoma [4]. Surgery of cerebellar haemangioblastomas is the basic treatment. However, serious complications are described. The main cause of postoperative death is bleeding to the brain stem and the remaining portions of the tumor [6]. Moreover, after surgical treatment, distant recurrences cannot be prevented [9]. There are only few studies on radiosurgery for haemangioblastomas with either the stereotactic linear accelerator [1, 2, 10, 14] or the Leksell gamma knife [5, 8, 11, 12]. The impact of radiosurgery for the treatment of cerebellar haemangioblastomas remains to be defined. This paper is an attempt to summarize the current knowledge of Gamma Knife surgery (GKS) for cerebellar haemangioblastomas. A review of the literature is compared to the results obtained in Munich during a 10-year-period of outpatient GKS for this special indication.

Patients and results

A total of 23 haemangioblastomas were treated in 11 individuals with 17 GKS sessions. Median age was 47 years (range: 17–59). All patients had a Karnofsky performance score (KPS) between 70 and 100 (median KPS: 80). Two patients were female. Two patients had sporadic haemangioblastomas, nine von Hippel Lindau syndrome. Two patients had lesions in the Medulla oblongata. Eight patients had one to three microsurgical resections before GKS. No patient received fractionated radiation therapy before or after GKS. Median dose prescribed to the tumor margin was 18 Gy (range: 14–20). The median isodose at the tumor magin was 50% (range: 50–80%). The median number of isocenters used per patient were five (range 1–14). In three patients a transient, asymptomatic swelling of treated tumors was detected after GKS. In one patient a cyst developed after GKS which had to be surgically aspirated. All other tumors could be controlled by radiosurgery alone. Patients with VHL disease tended to present with neurological symptoms and signs at a younger age than patients with sporadic disease ($p = 0.09$), presented with multiple lesions (53%), and developed new lesions (rate: 1 lesion/2.1 years).

Discussion

Treatment of symptomatic haemangioblastomas remains mainly neurosurgical, often in emergency, but stereotactic radiosurgery is emerging as an alternative therapeutic procedure [13]. Multiple haemangioblastomas of the central nervous system and retina are associated with von Hippel-Lindau disease and also predispose individuals to renal cell carcinomas and visceral cysts. In VHL, microsurgery or radiosurgery cannot prevent new haemangioblastomas from arising in the central nervous system [9]. Surgical outcomes for patients with CNS haemangioblastomas are favorable. However, they present management challenges due to their variable nature. They may be solid or cystic, solitary or multiple. Their vascularity and critical sites of origin often make complete resection impossible. Management of haemangioblastomas is even a more difficult and prolonged endeavor for patients with VHL syndrome. Routine neuroradiological screening is of particular importance and allows identification of lesions before they become symptomatic. Because patients with VHL syndrome are at risk for development of new lesions, they require lifelong follow-up [3].

The combined follow-up data of the 23 haemangioblastomas in 15 patients from the previous literature and the present series indicate that, first, a solitary

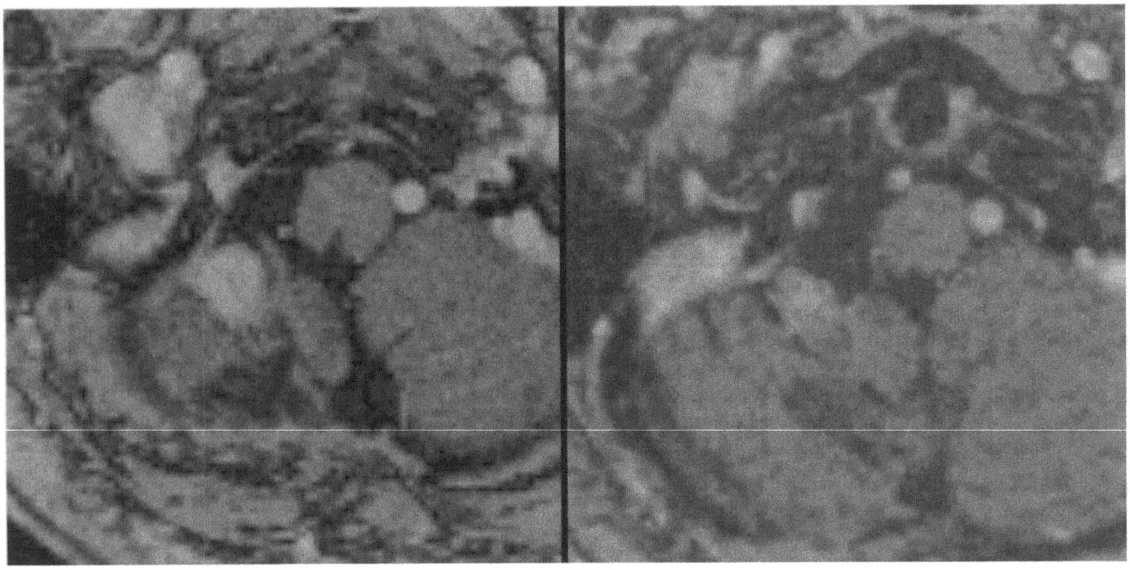

Fig. 1. Capillary cerebellar haemangioblastoma in the right cerebellar hemisphere (left image). Six years follow up after Gamma Knife Surgery demonstrates local tumor control and partial tumor shrinkage

small- or medium-sized haemangioblastoma usually shrinks or stops growing after radiosurgery. The recommended margin dose is 10 to 15 Gy. Second, the adjoining cyst often does not respond to radiosurgery but requires later, sometimes repeated evacuation [8]. The histopathological findings in these patients showed varying degrees of small vessel thickening and occlusion together with loss of tumor cells. The observations varied in degree according to the time between gamma knife radiosurgery and the secondary operation. These findings indicate the effectiveness of the treatment. The reduction in vascularity suggests that gamma knife radiosurgery could make subsequent surgery less hazardous. Pan *et al.* state that while radiosurgery is not adequately reliable for the control of haemangioblastoma cysts, it is an effective treatment for solid tumors and may be an alternative to surgery for those tumors located in eloquent regions [11]. The multicenter trial of Parice *et al.* [12] documents the largest experience in the literature (38 tumors) using stereotactic radiosurgery for the treatment of cerebellar haemangioblastoma. He found an 86% actuarial rate of tumor control at two years. Similar results have been reported by other authors and match the results of our series [2, 8, 12].

Conclusion

We conclude according to our experience and the data from the literature: (a) haemangioblastomas are particularly amenable to radiosurgery because they are often small, well delineated, and contain susceptible vascular elements, (b) radiosurgery controls the majority of primary and recurrent haemangioblastomas; (c) radiosurgery offers the ability to treat multiple lesions in a single treatment session, which is particularly important for patients with von Hippel-Lindau Syndrome where resection of multiple tumors might be precluded because of brain location; and that (d) better control rates are associated with higher radiosurgical doses and smaller tumor volumes.

References

1. Chakraborti PR, Chakrabarti KB, Doughty D, Plowman PN (1997) Stereotactic multiple are radiotherapy. IV – Haemangioblastoma. Br J Neurosurg 11: 110–115
2. Chang SD, Meisel JA, Hancock SL, Martin DP, McManus M, Adler JR Jr (1998) Treatment of haemangioblastomas in von Hippel-Lindau disease with linear accelerator-based radiosurgery. Neurosurgery 43: 28–34; discussion 34–25
3. Conway JE, Chou D, Clatterbuck RE, Brem H, Long DM, Rigamonti D (2001) Haemangioblastomas of the central nervous system in von Hippel-Lindau syndrome and sporadic disease. Neurosurgery 48: 55–62; discussion 62–53
4. Decq P (1998) [Guidelines for the maintenance of Hippel-Lindau disease in daily practice. French Society of Neurosurgery]. Neurochirurgie 44: 273–274
5. Georg AE, Lunsford LD, Kondziolka D, Flickinger JC, Maitz A (1997) Haemangioblastoma of the posterior fossa. The role of multimodality treatment. Arq Neuropsiquiatr 55: 278–286
6. Maddock IR, Moran A, Maher ER, Teare MD, Norman A, Payne SJ, Whitehouse R, Dodd C, Lavin M, Hartley N, Super M, Evans DG (1996) A genetic register for von Hippel-Lindau disease. J Med Genet 33: 120–127

7. Maher ER, Iselius L, Yates JR, Littler M, Benjamin C, Harris R, Sampson J, Williams A, Ferguson-Smith MA, Morton N (1991) Von Hippel-Lindau disease: a genetic study. J Med Genet 28: 443–447
8. Niemel M, Lim YJ, Soderman M, Jaaskelainen J, Lindquist C (1996) Gamma knife radiosurgery in 11 haemangioblastomas. J Neurosurg 85: 591–596
9. Niemela M, Maenpaa H, Salven P, Summanen P, Poussa K, Laatikainen L, Jaaskelainen J, Joensuu H (2001) Interferon alpha-2a therapy in 18 haemangioblastomas. Clin Cancer Res 7: 510–516
10. Page KA, Wayson K, Steinberg GK, Adler JR Jr (1993) Stereotaxic radiosurgical ablation: an alternative treatment for recurrent and multifocal haemangioblastomas. A report of four cases. Surg Neurol 40: 424–428
11. Pan L, Wang EM, Wang BJ, Zhou LF, Zhang N, Cai PW, Da JZ (1998) Gamma knife radiosurgery for haemangioblastomas. Stereotact Funct Neurosurg 70 [Suppl] 1: 179–186
12. Patrice SJ, Sneed PK, Flickinger JC, Shrieve DC, Pollock BE, Alexander E 3rd, Larson DA, Kondziolka DS, Gutin PH, Wara WM, McDermott MW, Lunsford LD, Loeffler JS (1996) Radiosurgery for haemangioblastoma: results of a multi-institutional experience. Int J Radiat Oncol Biol Phys 35: 493–499
13. Richard S, David P, Marsot-Dupuch K, Giraud S, Beroud C, Resche F (2000) Central nervous system haemangioblastomas, endolymphatic sac tumors, and von Hippel-Lindau disease. Neurosurg Rev 23: 1–22; discussion 23–24
14. Sawin PD, Follett KA, Wen BC, Laws ER Jr (1996) Symptomatic intrasellar haemangioblastoma in a child treated with subtotal resection and adjuvant radiosurgery. Case report. J Neurosurg 84: 1046–1050
15. Zbar B, Kaelin W, Maher E, Richard S (1999) Third International Meeting on von Hippel-Lindau disease. Cancer Res 59: 2251–2253

4. Meningeal hemangiopericytoma

Summary

Meningeal hemangiopericytoma represents a rare indication of Gamma Knife Surgery. Small remnants after surgical debulking or tumor recurrences are mainly treated. There is no indication for upfront radiosurgery because (semi)malignant hemangiopericytoma is undistinguishable from benign meningioma based on imaging appearance alone. The therapeutic profile of outpatient Gamma Knife Surgery is characterized by a high local tumor control, the possibility of radiosurgical salvage treatment and low treatment related morbidity. Radiosurgery is superior to whole brain therapy in respect of long term efficacy and side effects.

Keywords: Gamma knife surgery; hemangiopericytoma; radiosurgery.

Introduction

Haemangiopericytoma (HPC) is a rare, highly cellular and richly vascularized brain tumor (WHO grade II or III) almost always attached to the dura with a tendency to recur and metastasize outside the central nervous system (CNS) [8]. The incidence is approximately 0.4% of all primary brain tumors with a ratio of HPC to meningioma of about 1 : 50 [9]. The tumors are very similar to meningiomas with respect to their appearance on computed tomography (CT) and magnetic resonance imaging (MRI). Therefore a histological examination is mandatory for correct diagnosis of HPC and neurosurgical resection remains first line therapy in all patients [3, 12]. In this paper we try to define the contribution of radiosurgery to the therapeutic armoury for recurrent HPC. A review of the radiosurgical literature is given and the results obtained in Munich during a 10-year-period of outpatient gamma knife radiosurgery for HPC are analysed.

Patients and results

Within a 10-year-period ten patients received eleven Gamma Knife surgical (GKS) sessions for HPC (Table 1). In two patients, two lesions were treated in one session. The total number of treated HPC lesions were thirteen. This represents 0.4% of all GKS procedures in our centre. The reason for a second GKS was a new distant HPC in one patient. One patient had chemotherapy before GKS because of multiple extracranial metastases. Another patient had tumor embolisation prior to surgery for HPC. Four patients were irradiated by conventional radiotherapy before GKS. All patients had one to three neurosurgical tumor resections before GKS. Median age was 53.9 years (28.6–70.0). The targets of GKS were small HPC recurrences in all cases. The median tumor volume was calculated to 5.2 cm^3 (1.4 cm^3–26.7 cm^3). The lesions were exposed to a median dose to the tumor margin of 19.8 Gy (16 Gy–20 Gy). This corresponded to a peripheral isodose of 50% (50%–60%). Documented by MRI and clinical examination, the median follow-up time was 9.9 (2.7–42.6) months after GKS. All tumors were controlled after radiosurgery (Fig. 1). In one patient MRI showed a transient flare of gadolinium two years after GKS. This imaging change was not correlated to neurological symptoms. Symptomatic neurological side effects of GKS were not observed. One patient needed resection of a recurrent HPC that was too large for GKS.

Discussion

The majority of HPC can be removed by microsurgery in a seemingly complete manner but local recurrences are almost inevitable in the long run [8, 10]. Moreover, total excision often cannot be achieved when haemangiopericytomas arise from the skull base or involve the venous sinuses. This could also be confirmed in the present patient series. All patients had local recurrences after previous microsurgical resection. Because of the recurrent nature of these lesions, external-beam radiotherapy has been used in the postoperative setting. Postoperative radiotherapy and/or chemotherapy increase patient survival time and reduce local recurrences [1, 2, 5, 11, 14, 15]. Radiation

Table 1. *Characteristics and treatment data of ten HPC patients treated by GKS*

	HPC patients	With radiotherapy	Without radiotherapy	Significance
Sex				
Female/male	8/2			
Age	27.5 (9.5–57.6)			
Karnofsky performance score	70 (60–100)			
Neurological deficit before GKS	9			
Fractionated radiotherapy	4			
Surgical interventions	10 (1–3 per pat)			
Interval				
1. Surgery – GKS (y)	4 (2–11)	3.2 ± 1.2	8.5 ± 11	P < 0.02
Tumor localization				
Treatment parameters				
Tumor volume (cm^3)	5.2 (1.4–26.7)			
Tumor dose (D_{min}, Gy)	19.8 (16–20)			
No. of isocentres	10 (3–20)			
Peripheral isodose (%)	50 (50–60)			
Outcome after GKS				
Radiation toxicity	1 asympt.		1 asympt.	
Recurrence after GKS	1 distant (OP)			

Table 2. *Radiosurgical series for HPC*

Author	No. of patients	No. of lesions (2nd RS)	Study period (years)	Previous surgery	Fractionated Radiotherapy
Coffey	5	11 (2)		100%	3 (60%)
Galanis	10	20	20	100%	7 (70%)
Payne	12	15			
Sheehan	14	15	14	100%	7 (50%)
Chang	8	8	10	100%	5 (63%)
Wowra	10	12 (1)	10	100%	4 (40%)
Summary	54	70 (3)	10–20	100%	

The first report of Coffey *et al.* is included in the series of Galanis *et al.*

responses are dose dependent, with >50 Gy providing superior long-term disease-free survival [1, 2, 14]. However, it could not be demonstrated that postoperative radiotherapy can protect the neuraxis or peripheral metastasis [5]. After 15 years a recurrence rate between 85% and 91% has been reported [4, 6, 7, 13, 16]. These findings correspond well to our experience. The median time after surgery to gamma knife radiosurgery was four years. Radiation therapy after surgery extended the average time to the first gamma knife procedure from three years to eight years in the present series. The well defined nature of these lesions on MR imaging, however, makes them attractive targets for stereotactic radiosurgery (Tables 2, 3). Radiosurgery may be regarded as a means of local dose escalation with two further advantages over fractionated radiotherapy. The first is that it is possible to deliver a high, effective dose to the tumor and to keep the dose to healthy tissue to a minimum. This also implies the possibility to apply radiosurgery even after full dose fractionated radiotherapy. The second advantage is that GKS may be given repeatedly for distant recurrences. However, radiosurgery is a focal treatment and does not necessarily prevent regional and distant metastases. The aggressive nature of hemangiopericytomas can result in initial decreases in tumor size to be followed by later regrowth [12]. Therefore, the need for close clinical and radiographic follow-up observation in this patient population is of particular importance.

Conclusion

Neurosurgical resection remains the first line treatment for haemangiopericytoma. Only by surgery the histology of these rare lesions can be ascertained and mass reduction can be accomplished if necessary. The evidenced data base supports a very favourable role of radiosurgery for residual or recurrent haemangiopericytoma after surgery. Salvage radiosurgery is a powerful tool to treat new distant haemangiopericytoma recurrences repeatedly when they evolve. There are some arguments in favour of higher radiosurgical dose between 17 and 20 Gy directed to the tumor margin. Because of the rarity of these lesions however, sound statistics to support this opinion are not available. Even though some tumors undergo complete regression, there remains a need for life-long

Table 3. *Radiosurgical series for HPC*

Author	Device	Dose (D_{min}, Gy)	Follow up (mo)	Local control	Deaths Related to HPC	Side effects of radiosurgery
Coffey	LGK			100%		
Galanis	LGK	(12–18)		100%		
Payne	LGK	14 (2.8–25)	24.8	67%		
Sheehan	LGK	15 (11–20)	31.3	80%		
Chang	LCK	20.8 (16–24)	44	75%		
Wowra	LGK	19.8 (16–20)	10	100%		1 As RT
Summary						

The first report of Coffey [4] is included in the series of Galanis [6].
LGK Leksell gamma knife; *L* stereotactic Linac; *CK* Cyber knife, *mo* months, *As* asymptomatic, *RT* radiation toxicity.

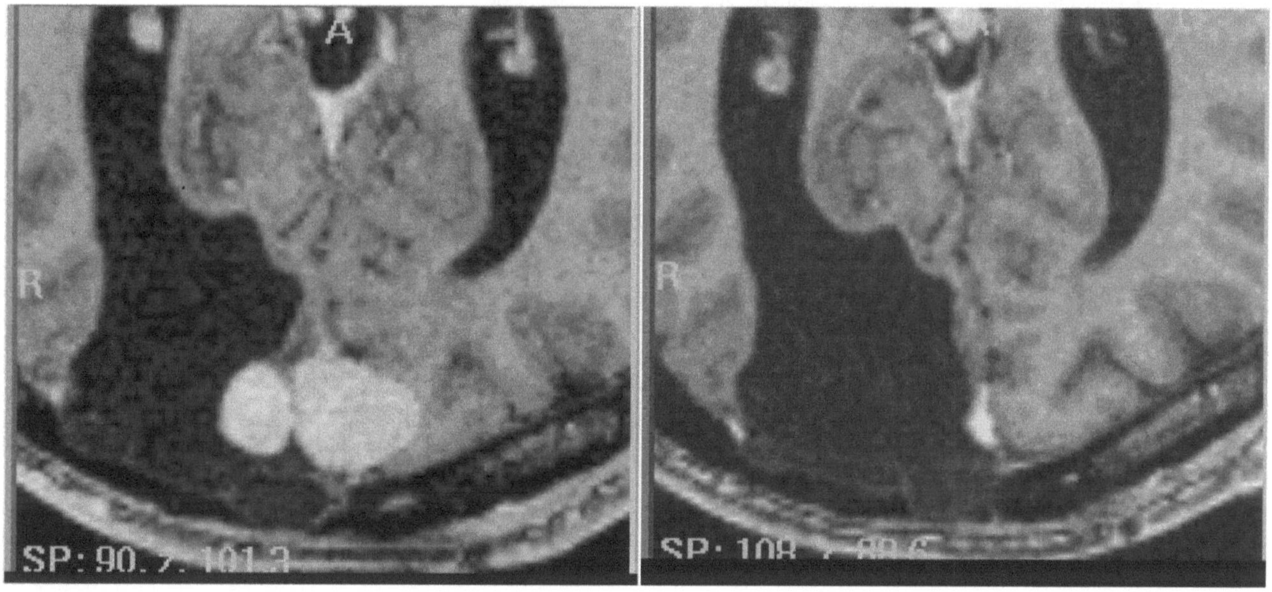

Fig. 1. Malignant haemangiopericytoma WHO grade III: Local recurrence after microsurgical resection right occipital tumor (left image). Complete remission 1.5 years after Gamma Knife Radiosurgery (right image)

MRI surveillance of affected individuals. Side effects of radiosurgery are moderate making gamma knife radiosurgery together with the high local tumor control rates a valuable neurosurgical tool for residual or recurrent haemangiopericytoma.

References

1. Bastin KT, Mehta MP (1992) Meningeal hemangiopericytoma: defining the role for radiation therapy. J Neurooncol 14: 277–287
2. Borg MF, Benjamin CS (1994) A 20-year review of haemangiopericytoma in Auckland, New Zealand. Clin Oncol (R Coll Radiol) 6: 371–376
3. Chang SD, Sakamoto GT (2003) The role of radiosurgery for hemangiopericytoma. Neurosurg Focus 14: 1–5
4. Coffey RJ, Cascino TL, Shaw EG (1993) Radiosurgical treatment of recurrent hemangiopericytomas of the meninges: preliminary results. J Neurosurg 78: 903–908
5. Dufour H, Metellus P, Fuentes S, Murracciole X, Regis J, Figarella-Branger D, Grisoli F (2001) Meningeal hemangiopericytoma: a retrospective study of 21 patients with special review of postoperative external radiotherapy. Neurosurgery 48: 756–762; discussion 762–753
6. Galanis E, Buckner JC, Scheithauer BW, Kimmel DW, Schomberg PJ, Piepgras DG (1998) Management of recurrent meningeal hemangiopericytoma. Cancer 82: 1915–1920
7. Guthrie BL, Ebersold MJ, Scheithauer BW, Shaw EG (1989) Meningeal hemangiopericytoma: histopathological features, treatment, and long-term follow-up of 44 cases. Neurosurgery 25: 514–522
8. Jääskeläinen J, Louis DN, Paulus W, Plate KH, Haltia MJ (1997) Haemangiopericytoma. In: Kleihues P, Cavenee WK (eds) Pathology and genetics of tumors of the nervous system. International Agency for Research on Cancer, Lyon, pp 146–148
9. Jääskelainen J, Servo A, Haltia M, Wahlstrom T, Valtonen S

(1985) Intracranial hemangiopericytoma: radiology, surgery, radiotherapy, and outcome in 21 patients. Surg Neurol 23: 227–236
10. Kim JH, Jung HW, Kim YS, Kim CJ, Hwang SK, Paek SH, Kim DG, Kwun BD (2003) Meningeal hemangiopericytomas: long-term outcome and biological behavior. Surg Neurol 59: 47–53; discussion 53–44
11. Mena H, Ribas JL, Pezeshkpour GH, Cowan DN, Parisi JE (1991) Hemangiopericytoma of the central nervous system: a review of 94 cases. Hum Pathol 22: 84–91
12. Payne B, Prasad D, Steiner M, Steiner L (2000) Gamma surgery for hemangiopericytomas. Acta Neurochir (Wien) 142: 527–536; discussion 536–527
13. Sheehan J, Kondziolka D, Flickinger J, Lunsford LD (2002) Radiosurgery for treatment of recurrent intracranial hemangiopericytomas. Neurosurgery 51: 905–910; discussion 910–901
14. Someya M, Sakata KI, Oouchi A, Nagakura H, Satoh M, Hareyama M (2001) Four cases of meningeal hemangiopericytoma treated with surgery and radiotherapy. Jpn J Clin Oncol 31: 548–552
15. Soyuer S, Chang EL, Selek U, McCutcheon IE, Maor MH (2004) Intracranial meningeal hemangiopericytoma: the role of radiotherapy: report of 29 cases and review of the literature. Cancer 100: 1491–1497
16. Vuorinen V, Sallinen P, Haapasalo H, Visakorpi T, Kallio M, Jaaskelainen J (1996) Outcome of 31 intracranial haemangiopericytomas: poor predictive value of cell proliferation indices. Acta Neurochir (Wien) 138: 1399–1408

Correspondence: Dr. Berndt Wowra, Gamma Knife Center, Ingolstädter Str. 166, 80939 Munich, Germany. e-mail: wowra@gammaknife.de

Acta Neurochir (2004) [Suppl] 91: 103–108

Microneurosurgery and radiosurgery – an attractive combination

J.-C. Tonn

Department of Neurosurgery, Maximilians University, Munich, Germany

Summary

Microneurosurgery and radiosurgery have made tremendous progress in terms of increasing efficacy and reducing treatment related mobility. Both techniques have clear indications; however, there is still competition between the two modalities in a variety of diseases. In all instances, this rivalry should be replaced by the concept of using both methods as complementary. Skull base tumours, metastases as well as certain AVMs are good candidates for this approach.

Keywords: Microneurosurgery; radiosurgery; meningioma; neurinoma; skull base tumours; AVM; brain metastases; gamma knife.

Introduction

The outstanding advances in microneurosurgery, induced by technical developments in diagnostics and the supportive equipment in the operation theatre, all serve the issue "nihil nocere". Main priority is given to the preservation of integrity and function of the CNS. Knowledge of the natural courses and etiology as well as the pathogenesis of diseases is growing continuously and generates the wish to find a treatment modality as causal as possible and least invasive for the organism. Hence the concept of "minimally invasive" therapy was formed – ideally combining maximum therapeutic efficiency with minimal strain on the patient. Today this concept is not only exposed to an evaluation of efficiency in the sense of evidenced based medicine, there is also the demand for an economic and target oriented use of medico-economic resources becoming ever more restricted. Not just the actual costs of treatment have to be calculated but also the economic costs caused by treatment induced morbidity have to be taken into account. Seen from these points of view debates on radio- and microneurosurgery as being procedures excluding each other and competing against each other appear to be anachronistic. The present paper is meant to be an invitation to regard the two methods as complementary.

Meningiomas

The prognosis of patients with meningiomas is essentially determined by their histologic grading and localization of the tumour. Over 90% of the tumours are classified into WHO grade 1 (rarely grade 2), while histologic subtypes among grade 1 tumours have no prognostic value [13]. More decisive are localization and extension of the lesion: meningiomas of the skull base show much higher recurrence rates – for meningiomas involving the orbit this rate is over 40%. This is due to the fact that for anatomical reasons a radical resection (corresponding to Simpson Grade I) is possible only in selected cases. Also, the risk of treatment induced morbidity when microsurgically removing large skull base meningiomas is significantly increased. From this two general guidelines for the indication and selection of treatment modality can be deduced:

1) For *symptomatic* meningiomas treatment should in general begin as early as possible, i.e. at a time point of smallest extension. Especially for skull base meningiomas microsurgical extirpation is best possible in cases of favourable prognostic factors corresponding to Simpson grades I and II. Also, the minor involvement of cerebral nerves and vessel structures of the skull base as seen in smaller tumours offers a gentle removal with low risk of morbidity. The same applies to meningiomas invading the venous sinus. Here an early removal under resection of the outer dural sheath at the sinus is often possible and allows complete resection without necessity of sinus reconstruction [18].

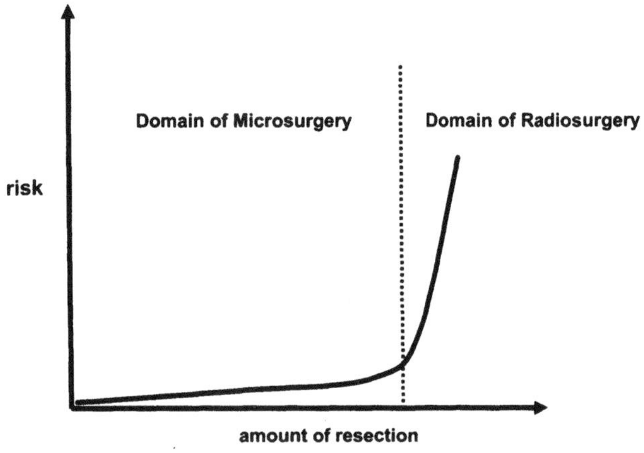

Fig. 1. Graphic illustration of the relation "amount of resection versus risk". The domain of microneurosurgery comprehends the extensive resection at low risk. In case of dramatic increase of the surgical risk profile, albeit very small additional resection feasibility, radiosurgery should be considered for these remnants

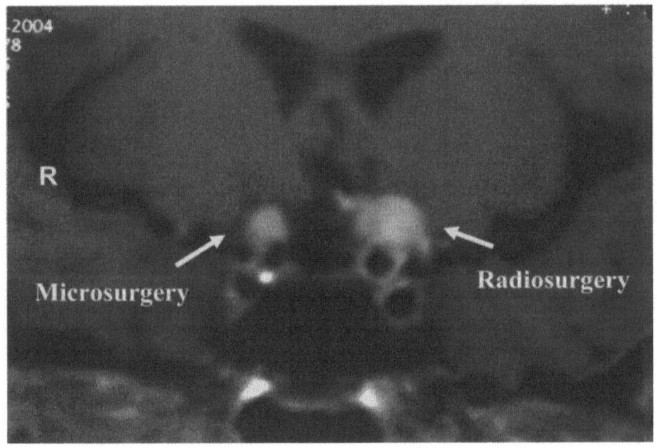

Fig. 2. Recurrent meningioma, bilaterally. Left eye: amarosis; right eye: dramatic visual deterioration. Due to close proximity of the right tumour to the optic nerve with entrapment of the optic nerve within the optic canal by the tumour, radiosurgery was considered for the left and microneurosurgical decompression for the right side

For smaller skull base meningiomas, radiosurgery is an alternative to the microsurgical approach. Therapists today should offer this method to the patient when informing him, presented by the respective specialist for each treatment modality (in mutual agreement). Here again the same rationale applies: in light of radiotherapeutic/radio-biologic considerations a small tumour volume and hence an early treatment is most effective and least invasive (see chapter in this book).

For *asymptomatic* meningiomas, diagnosed mostly by chance, regular MRI controls should be undertaken (initially at 6 months, then yearly) under comparable technical conditions. When radiology demonstrates growth, indication for treatment is given, also when symptoms associated with the tumour occur, even if size of the lesion remains constant.

2) For large tumours it is necessary to optimise the ratio of resection radicality to therapy induced morbidity to achieve best possible treatment results:

$$\textit{Equation}\text{: Quality} = \frac{\text{resection radicality}}{\text{therapy induced morbidity}}$$

Especially in cases of large, complex skull base meningiomas (for example large petroclival meningiomas, meningiomas involving the superior orbital fissure and cavernous sinus, cranio-cervical meningiomas with extensive ventral tumour base), not seldom after considerable microsurgical size reduction with extensive dissection, the risk of functional damage increases exponentially from a certain point of the procedure.

In this case, the phase of surgery has to be chosen carefully during the operation from which radiosurgical therapy of the now significantly reduced tumour residue would be the better treatment option: a reduction in size improves considerably preconditions for radiosurgery and the threat of direct compression of functionally important structures (for example brain stem, hypothalamus, chiasm) is considerably reduced or eliminated. Furthermore radiosurgery avoids the operative danger which at that phase is great so that a combination of the two treatment modalities would assure the high therapeutic quotient aimed at [2, 6, 7, 9, 12, 25].

The following constellations are particularly suitable for a combined treatment (extensive resection and removal of the mass-effect as pre-requirement for radiosurgical treatment of the tumour base):

- Petroclival meningiomas with supratentorial extension, invading the cavernous sinus
- Petroclival meningiomas encircling the basilar artery and their pontine perforators
- Meningiomas of the cranio-cervical transition with ventral tumour base and enveloping the caudal cranial nerves
- Meningiomas involving the cavernous sinus (radiosurgery of the intracavernous part) [4, 11, 14, 15, 19, 20, 21, 30]

- Meningiomas of the parasellar region invading the cavernous sinus and the superior orbital fissure (microsurgical resection of those parts compressing the optic nerve/the chiasm in order to maintain visual acuity and to gain distance of the radiation target volume from the optic system
- Parts of medial sphenoid wing meningiomas which have surrounded the carotid artery in the region of the perforating branches supplying the basal ganglia (these residues should only be treated radiosurgically when progression of the remaining tumour is proven. (Close follow-up magnetic resonance process controls are mandatory.)
- Parasagittal meningiomas under inclusion of the perfused filled superior sagittal sinus and the bridging veins (tumour reduction under preservation of the veins ending there, radiosurgery when tumour progresses).
- For all intrameatal portions of tumour (for example optic canal, internal auditory canal), subtle microsurgical decompression has to be preferred over radiosurgical treatment because radiation induced increase of volume (swelling) may cause additional damage. Especially tumour parts at/in the optic canal have to be decompressed/removed since the vicinity to the optic canal with its reduced radiation tolerance implies a high functional risk. However, surgical intervention in this area demands extensive surgical expertise.

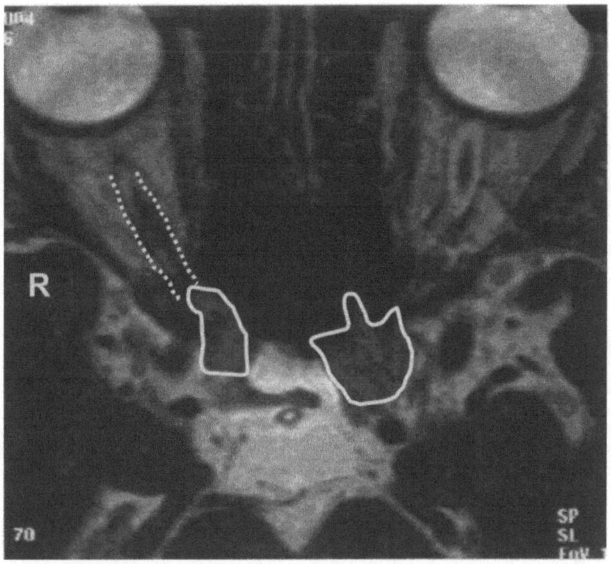

Fig. 3. Tumour (solid line), and optic nerve (dotted line) with tumour extension into the right optic canal

Intracranial neurinomas

Microsurgical treatment of acoustic neurinomas today is performed in centres with high frequency of acoustic neurinoma operations per year at a very high standard. The rate of hearing preservation in patients with a preoperatively functionally usable hearing is 50–60%. Permanent pareses of the facial nerve occur in approx. 10–14% of cases, rates of high grade facial palsy/plegia are very low (below 5%) [17, 27–29, 33]. However, demands from patients and referring physicians to preserve function and maintain hearing are rising. Here microsurgery and radiosurgery compete against each other. Especially large acoustic neurinomas with brain stem compression should still be treated microsurgically in order to anticipate the danger of a further brain stem compression (induced by growth or radiogenous swelling). In cases of tumour/capsule fragments adjacent to the cranial nerves which are very difficult to be resected from the cranial nerves (and only with significantly increased functional risk for nerve functions) it is recommendable to leave these residues untreated. Regular MRI controls should be performed (recommended yearly). Progression rate of such intentionally left residues is given as 8–20% [32]. If the tumour continues to grow, radiosurgery should be preferred since already in the first instance complete removal was considered too risky [22, 23]. For "genuine" tumour recurrences with no initial residue left, recurrence rates lie between 1–9%. A decision as to which treatment approach to be chosen for the recurrent tumour should be made individually.

From our own experience it cannot be confirmed that pre-radiated tumours are more difficult to operate.

With regard to trigeminal schwannomas similar viewpoints apply for the selection and indication of therapies [5, 10]. In patients with trigeminal neuropathy due to direct irritation (compression), microsurgical decompression eliminates rapidly the pain syndrome. Usually this is what ultimately matters most to the patient. Also, a so-called "pain memory" is avoided if the time span for pain anamnesis is kept short.

Hypophyseal tumours

Indication for the treatment of hypophyseal tumours depends on their size (for example compression

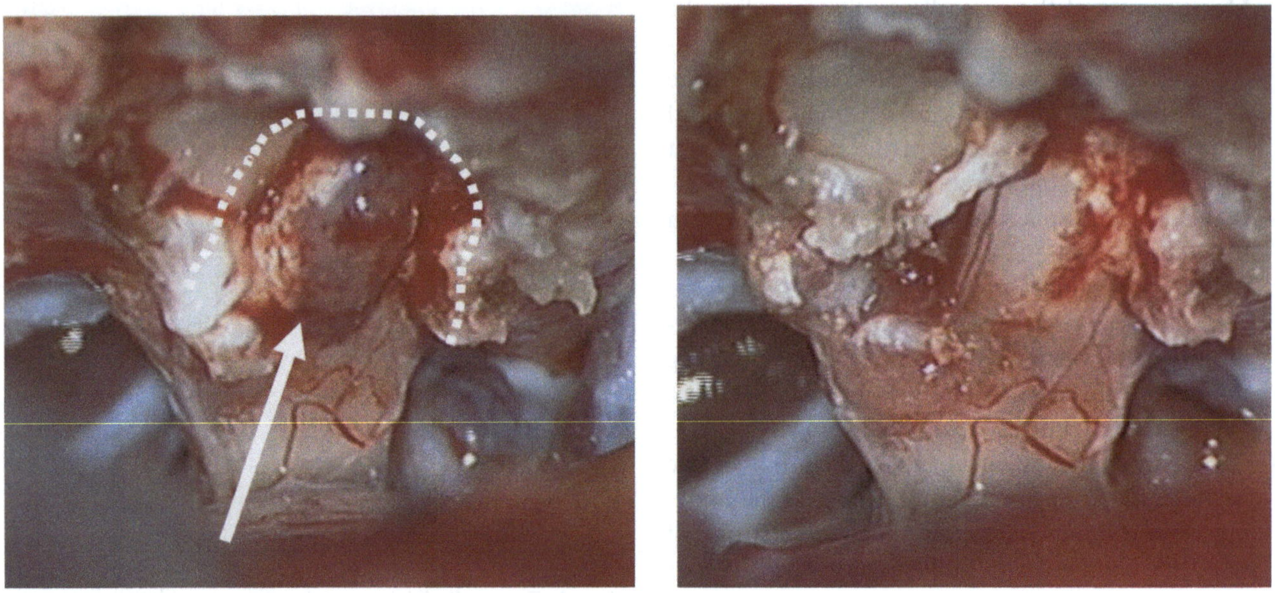

Fig. 4. *Left*: after unroofing of the optic canal (dotted line), the tumour within the canal was exposed (arrow). *Right*: optic nerve after tumour resection

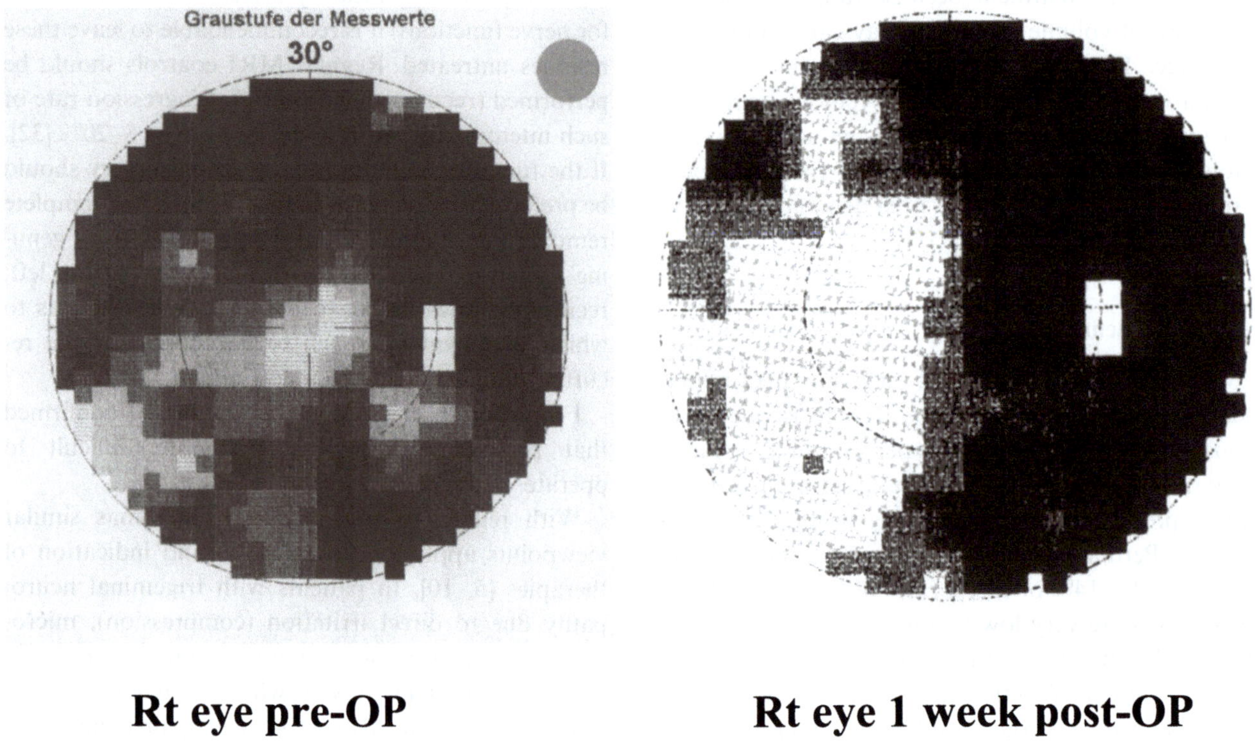

Fig. 5. Visual field of right eye prior to (left) and after (right) surgery. Vision improved from 0.1 to 0.4

of the chiasm, optic nerve, compression of the hypothalamus, brain stem, etc.) and/or autonomous hormone production. Correspondingly, decrease of volume and decompression or removal of a hormone secreting adenoma are the therapeutic goals that can be achieved rapidly and at low risk by surgery. Invasively growing adenoma parts, especially with extension towards the cavernous sinus, often evade complete resection. Here tight meshed, regular controls are necessary in order to early detect progression of the residue. Not before then is the indication for radiosurgery given as many adenoma residues remain stationary for long even without adjuvant therapy. If radiosurgery is indicated for large invasive adenomas/adenoma residues, it has to be determined in each case whether microsurgical resection of those parts close to the chiasm/optic nerve is required to make sure that the radiation target volumes are in a safe distance to radiation sensible structures. Modern hypophyseal surgery must assure that the function of the optic system as well as the structures of the cavernous sinus and the endocrinologic function of the hypophyseal frontal and posterior lobe be maintained. This can be achieved through a combination of subtle micro-neurosurgical and radiosurgical procedures (see chapter in this book).

Metastasis

Radiosurgical management of brain metastases today is the accepted standard treatment. Also in cases of so-called radiation resistant tumours good results can be achieved. The operative therapy has its domain in the extirpation of space occupying lesions with a diameter of >3.5 cm. Surgical resection of large space occupying metastases combined with radiosurgy of further small ones, also in patients with multiple metastases, offers good outcomes, provided the patient is in a good general state and has a favourable prognosis in relation to the basic disease. The results of a current randomised study on open microsurgery versus gamma knife radiosurgery of single brain metastases are still outstanding.

In individual cases it may be required to surgically remove radiogenous necrosis after radiosurgical therapy if space occupying edema or epileptic seizures can no longer be treated conservatively.

AVM

For arteriovenous malformations several therapeutical options are available which have to be used in combination in a considerable number of patients [31]. Endovascular embolization and surgical resection remain to be the most efficient and, especially in combination, safest approach in terms of controlling the risk of recurrent haemorrhages in lesions that have bled. However, sometimes small remnants are resectable only with a significant risk of surgical morbidity. These, and small, deep seated AVMs are suitable targets for radiosurgical approaches [3, 16]. A meticulous analysis of risk factors, treatment related as well as in relation to the natural history, is mandatory [1, 16]. In any case, each patient has to be treated in a multidisciplinary approach from the very beginning [31].

Cavernomas are no suitable target for radiosurgery since surgical procedures are safe and effective in terms of prevention of recurrent haemorrhages as well as seizure control. Developmental venous anomalies (DVA), formerly called "venous angiomas", are not subject of any treatment whatsoever since they are an indispensable element of the venous drainage.

Conclusion

Micro-neurosurgery and radiosurgery are complementary in many ways. An unbiased examination of treatment methods will open new ways of supplementary applications. By combining the advantages of the different therapies while accepting and jointly minimizing their inherent risks and limitations, treatment goals achieved in common will markedly be improved.

Prerequisites are

- Intensive communication and cooperation between microneurosurgeon and radiosurgeon
- joint concepts and consensus
- team effort
- mutual prospective documentation of results and failures, evaluation, (peer reviewed) publication of treatment results

Acknowledgment

The invaluable support by Mrs. I. Anders during preparation of this manuscript is highly appreciated.

References

1. Barker FG 2nd, Butler WE, Lyons S, Cascio E, Ogilvy CS, Loeffler JS, Chapman PH (2003) Dose-volume prediction of radiation-related complications after proton beam radiosurgery for cerebral arteriovenous malformations. J Neurosurg 99: 254–263
2. Biswas T, Sandhu AP, Singh DP, Schell MC, Maciunas RJ, Bakos RS, Muhs AG, Okunieff P (2003) Low-dose radiosurgery for benign intracranial lesions. Am J Clin Oncol 26: 325–331
3. Bollet MA, Anxionnat R, Buchheit I, Bey P, Cordebar A, Jay N, Desandes E, Marchal C, Lapeyre M, Aletti P, Picard L (2004) Efficacy and morbidity of arc-therapy radiosurgery for cerebral

arteriovenous malformations: a comparison with the natural history. Int J Radiat Oncol Biol Phys 58: 1353–1363
4. Chang SD, Adler JR Jr, Martin DP (1998) Linac radiosurgery for cavernous sinus meningiomas. Stereotact Funct Neurosurg 71: 43–50
5. Day JD, Fukushima T (1998) The surgical management of trigeminal neuromas. Neurosurgery 42: 233–241
6. Debus J, Wuendrich M, Pirzkall A, Hoess A, Schlegel W, Zuna I, Engenhart-Cabillic R, Wannenmacher M (2001) High efficacy of fractionated stereotactic radiotherapy of large base-of-skull meningiomas: long-term results. J Clin Oncol 19: 3547–3553
7. Dziuk TW, Woo S, Butler EB, Thornby J, Grossman R, Dennis WS, Lu H, Carpenter LS, Chiu JK (1998) Malignant meningiomas: an indication for initial aggressive surgery and adjuvant radiotherapy. J Neurooncol 37: 177–188
8. Fuss M, Debus J, Lohr F, Huber P, Rhein B, Engenhart-Cabillic R, Wannenmacher M (2000) Conventionally fractionated stereotactic radiotherapy (FSRT) for acoustic neuromas. Int J Radiat Oncol Biol Phys 48: 1381–1387
9. Harris AE, Lee JY, Omalu B, Flickinger JC, Kondziolka D, Lunsford LD (2003) The effect of radiosurgery during management of aggressive meningiomas. Surg Neurol 60: 298–305
10. Huang CF, Kondziolka D, Flickinger JC, Lunsford LD (1999) Stereotactic radiosurgery for trigeminal schwannomas. Neurosurgery 45: 11–16
11. Iwai Y, Yamanaka K, Ishiguro T (2003) Gamma knife radiosurgery for the treatment of cavernous sinus meningiomas. Neurosurgery 52: 517–524
12. Iwai Y, Yamanaka K, Nakajima H (2001) Two-staged gamma knife radiosurgery for the treatment of large petroclival and cavernous sinus meningiomas. Surg Neurol 56: 308–314
13. Kleihues P, Cavenee WK (eds) (2000) Pathology and genetics of tumours of the nervous system. WHO Classification of Tumours, IARC Press, Lyon
14. Kurita H, Sasaki T, Kawamoto S, Taniguchi M, Terahara A, Tago M, Kirino T (1997) Role of radiosurgery in the management of cavernous sinus meningiomas. Acta Neurol Scand 96: 297–304
15. Lee JY, Niranjan A, McInerney J, Kondziolka D, Flickinger JC, Lunsford LD (2002) Stereotactic radiosurgery providing long-term tumor control of cavernous sinus meningiomas. J Neurosurg 97: 65–72
16. Maruyama K, Kondziolka D, Niranjan A, Flickinger JC, Lunsford LD (2004) Stereotactic radiosurgery for brainstem arteriovenous malformations: factors affecting outcome. J Neurosurg 100: 407–413
17. Maw AR, Coakham HB, Ayoub O, Butler SR (2003) Hearing preservation and facial nerve function in vestibular schwannoma surgery. Clin Otolaryngol 28: 252–256
18. Mendenhall WM, Morris CG, Amdur RJ, Foote KD, Friedman WA (2003) Radiotherapy alone or after subtotal resection for benign skull base meningiomas. Cancer 98: 1473–1482
19. Nicolato A, Foroni R, Alessandrini F, Bricolo A, Gerosa M (2002) Radiosurgical treatment of cavernous sinus meningiomas: experience with 122 treated patients. Neurosurgery 51: 1153–1161
20. Nicolato A, Foroni R, Alessandrini F, Bricolo A, Gerosa M (2002) Radiosurgical treatment of cavernous sinus meningiomas: experience with 122 treated patients. Neurosurgery 2002 51: 1153–1161
21. Nicolato A, Foroni R, Alessandrini F, Maluta S, Bricolo A, Gerosa M (2002) The role of Gamma knife radiosurgery in the management of cavernous sinus meningiomas. Int J Radiat Oncol Biol Phys 53: 992–1000
22. Pellet W, Regis J, Roche PH, Delsanti C (2003) Relative indications for radiosurgery and microsurgery for acoustic schwannoma. Adv Tech Stand Neurosurg 28: 227–284
23. Pollock BE, Lunsford LD, Flickinger JC, Clyde BL, Kondziolka D (1998) Vestibular schwannoma management. Part I. Failed microsurgery and the role of delayed stereotactic radiosurgery. J Neurosurg 89: 944–948
24. Regis J, Pellet W, Delsanti C, Dufour H, Roche PH, Thomassin JM, Zanaret M, Peragut JC (2002) Functional outcome after gamma knife surgery or microsurgery for vestibular schwannomas. J Neurosurg 97: 1091–1100
25. Roche PH, Pellet W, Fuentes S, Thomassin JM, Regis J (2003) Gamma knife radiosurgical management of petroclival meningiomas, results and indications. Acta Neurochir 145: 883–888
26. Sakamoto T, Shirato H, Takeichi N, Aoyama H, Fukuda S, Miyasaka K (2001) Annual rate of hearing loss falls after fractionated stereotactic irradiation for vestibular schwannoma. Radiother Oncol 60: 45–48
27. Samii M, Matthies C (1997) Management of 1000 vestibular schwannomas (acoustic neuromas): surgical management and results with an emphasis on complications and how to avoid them. Neurosurgery 40: 11–23
28. Samii M, Matthies C (1997) Management of 1000 vestibular schwannomas (acoustic neuromas): the facial nerve – preservation and restitution of function. Neurosurgery 40: 684–695
29. Samii M, Matthies C (1997) Management of 1000 vestibular shwannomas (acoustic neuromas): hearing function in 1000 tumor resections. Neurosurgery 40: 248–262
30. Spiegelmann R, Nissim O, Menhel J, Alezra D, Pfeffer MR (2002) Linear accelerator radiosurgery for meningiomas in and around the cavernous sinus. Neurosurgery 51: 1373–1380
31. Steiger HJ, Schmid-Elsaesser R, Muacevic A, Brückmann H, Wowra B (eds) (2002) Neurosurgery of arteriovenous malformations and fistulas: a multimodal approach. Springer, Wien New York
32. Thomassin JM, Pellet W, Apron JP, Braccini F, Roche PH (2001) Recurrent acoustic neurinoma after complete surgical resection. Ann Otolaryngol Chir Cervicofac 118: 3–10
33. Tonn JC, Schlake HP, Goldbrunner R, Milewski C, Helms J, Roosen K (2000) Acoustic neuroma surgery as an interdisciplinary approach: a neurosurgical series of 508 patients. J Neurol Neurosurg Psychiatry 69: 161–166

Correspondence: Prof. Dr. J.-C. Tonn, Neurosurgical Department, Klinikum Großhadern, Marchioninistr. 15, 81377 Munich, Germany. e-mail: Joerg.Christian.Tonn@med.uni-muenchen.de

Author index

Index of keywords

SpringerMedizin

ADVANCES AND TECHNICAL STANDARDS IN NEUROSURGERY

Volume 29

2004. XIV, 304 pages. 101 figures, partly in colour.
Hardcover **EUR 125,–**
(Recommended retail price)
Net-price subject to local VAT.
ISBN 3-211-14027-1

Advances: Disorders of Consciousness: Anatomical and Physiological Mechanisms (J. L. Valatx) • Advances in Craniosynostosis Research and Management (J. Guimarães-Ferreira, J. Miguéns, C. Lauritzen)
Technical Standards: Preoperative Clinical Evaluation, Outline of Surgical Technique and Outcome in Temporal Lobe Epilepsy (A. Immonen, L. Jutila, R. Kälviäinen, E. Mervaala, K. Partanen, J. Partanen, R. Vanninen, A. Ylinen, I. Alafuzoff, L. Paljärvi, H. Hurskainen, J. Rinne, M. Puranen, M. Vapalahti) • Motor Evoked Potential Monitoring for Spinal Cord and Brain Stem Surgery (F. Sala, P. Lanteri, A. Bricolo) • Motor Evoked Potential Monitoring for the Surgery of Brain Tumours and Vascular Malformations. (G. Neuloh, J. Schramm) • Functional Neuronavigation and Intraoperative MRI (C. Nimsky, O. Ganslandt, R. Fahlbusch) • Surgical Anatomy of the Insula (M. Guenot, J. Isnard, M. Sindou)

Volume 30

2005. Approx. 300 pages. Approx. 100 figures, mostly in colour.
Hardcover **EUR 125,–**
(Recommended retail price)
Net-price subject to local VAT.
ISBN 3-211-21403-8

Advances: • Depolarisation phenomena in traumatic and ischaemic brain injury (A. J. Strong, R. Dardis) • What is magnetoencephalography and why it is relevant to neurosurgery? (F. H. Lopes da Silva) • Disorders of consciousness: Electrophysiological evaluation and prognosis (C. Fischer) • Neurobiology of olfaction including recovery of function following trauma (B. Landis, Th. Hummel, I Rodriguez, J. S. Lacroix)
Technical Standards: • Surgical anatomy for skin and bone flaps (H. D. Fournier, V. Delliere, J. B. Gourraud, Ph. Mercier) • Sacral neuromodulation in lower urinary tract dysfunction (J. R. Vignes, M. de Seze, E. Dobremez, P. A. Joseph, J. Guerin) • Endoscopy of the spine (E. Frank, M. Hunt) • Prophylactic antibiotics in neurosurgery: proof and convictions (G. C. Blomstedt) • Prevention and treatment of postoperative pain (A. Chiaretti, A. Langer) • Endoscopic III ventriculostomy in the treatment of hydrocephalus in paediatric patients (G. Cinalli, C. Di Rocco, L. Massimi, G. Tamburrini)

SpringerWienNewYork

P.O. Box 89, Sachsenplatz 4–6, 1201 Wien, Österreich, Fax +43.1.330 24 26, books@springer.at, **springer.at**
Haberstraße 7, 69126 Heidelberg, Deutschland, Fax +49.6221.345-4229, orders@springer.de, springer.de
P.O. Box 2485, Secaucus, NJ 07096-2485, USA, Fax +1.201.348-4505, orders@springer-ny.com, springeronline.com
Eastern Book Service, 3–13, Hongo 3-chome, Bunkyo-ku, Tokyo 113, Japan, Fax +81.3.38 18 08 64, orders@svt-ebs.co.jp
Preisänderungen und Irrtümer vorbehalten.

Springer and the Environment

WE AT SPRINGER FIRMLY BELIEVE THAT AN INTERnational science publisher has a special obligation to the environment, and our corporate policies consistently reflect this conviction.

WE ALSO EXPECT OUR BUSINESS PARTNERS – PRINTERS, paper mills, packaging manufacturers, etc. – to commit themselves to using environmentally friendly materials and production processes.

THE PAPER IN THIS BOOK IS MADE FROM NO-CHLORINE pulp and is acid free, in conformance with international standards for paper permanency.

MIX
Papier aus verantwortungsvollen Quellen
Paper from responsible sources
FSC® C105338

If you have any concerns about our products,
you can contact us on
ProductSafety@springernature.com

In case Publisher is established outside the EU,
the EU authorized representative is:
Springer Nature Customer Service Center GmbH
Europaplatz 3, 69115 Heidelberg, Germany

Printed by Libri Plureos GmbH
in Hamburg, Germany